Cloud-Based Benchmarking of Medical Image Analysis

Allan Hanbury · Henning Müller
Georg Langs
Editors

Cloud-Based Benchmarking of Medical Image Analysis

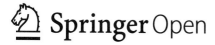

Editors
Allan Hanbury
Vienna University of Technology
Vienna
Austria

Georg Langs
Medical University of Vienna
Vienna
Austria

Henning Müller
University of Applied Sciences Western
  Switzerland
Sierre
Switzerland

ISBN 978-3-319-84207-3   ISBN 978-3-319-49644-3   (eBook)
DOI 10.1007/978-3-319-49644-3

Preface

The VISCERAL project[1] organized Benchmarks for analysis and retrieval of 3D medical images (CT and MRI) at a large scale. VISCERAL used an innovative cloud-based evaluation approach, where the image data were stored centrally on a cloud infrastructure, while participants placed their programs in virtual machines on the cloud. This way of doing evaluation will become increasingly important as evaluation of algorithms on increasingly large and potentially sensitive data that cannot be distributed will be done.

This book presents the points of view of both the organizers of the VISCERAL Benchmarks and the participants in these Benchmarks. The practical experience and knowledge gained in running such benchmarks in the new paradigm is presented by the organizers, while the participants report on their experiences with the evaluation paradigm from their point of view, as well as giving a description of the approaches submitted to the Benchmarks and the results obtained.

This book is divided into five parts. Part I presents the cloud-based benchmarking and Evaluation-as-a-Service paradigm that the VISCERAL Benchmarks used. Part II focusses on the datasets of medical images annotated with ground truth created in VISCERAL that continue to be available for research use, covering also the practical aspects of getting permission to use medical data and manually annotating 3D medical images efficiently and effectively. The VISCERAL Benchmarks are described in Part III, including a presentation and analysis of metrics used in the evaluation of medical image analysis and search. Finally, Parts IV and V present reports of some of the participants in the VISCERAL Benchmarks, with Part IV devoted to the Anatomy Benchmarks, which focused on segmentation and detection, and Part V devoted to the Retrieval Benchmark.

This book has two main audiences: *Medical Imaging Researchers* will be most interested in the actual segmentation, detection and retrieval results obtained for the tasks defined for the VISCERAL Benchmarks, as well as in the resources (annotated medical images and open source code) generated in the VISCERAL project,

---

[1] http://visceral.eu

while *eScience and Computational Science Reproducibility Advocates* will gain from the experience described in using the Evaluation-as-a-Service paradigm for evaluation and benchmarking on huge amounts of data.

Vienna, Austria   Allan Hanbury
Sierre, Switzerland   Henning Müller
Vienna, Austria   Georg Langs
September 2016

Acknowledgements

The work leading to the results presented in this book has received funding from the European Union Seventh Framework Programme (FP7/2007–2013) under Grant Agreement No. 318068 (VISCERAL).

The cloud infrastructure for the benchmarks was and continues to be supported by Microsoft Research on the Microsoft Azure Cloud.

We thank the reviewers of the VISCERAL project for their useful suggestions and advice on the project reviews. We also thank the VISCERAL EC Project Officer, Martina Eydner, for her support in efficiently handling the administrative aspects of the project.

We thank the many participants in the VISCERAL Benchmarks, especially those that participated in multiple Benchmarks. This enabled a very useful resource to be created for the medical imaging research community. We also thank all contributors to this book and the reviewers of the chapters (Marc-André Weber, Oscar Jimenez del Toro, Orcun Goksel, Adrien Depeursinge, Markus Krenn, Yashin Dicente, Johannes Hofmanninger, Peter Roth, Martin Urschler, Wolfgang Birkfellner, Antonio Foncubierta Rodríguez).

---

[1] http://visceral.eu

Contents

Contributors

Jennifer Alvén
Department of Signals and Systems, Chalmers University of Technology,
Gothenburg, Sweden
e-mail: alven@chalmers.se

Abdel Aziz Taha
Institute of Software Technology and Interactive Systems,
TU Wien, Vienna, Austria
e-mail: taha@ifs.tuwien.ac.at

Weidong Cai
Biomedical and Multimedia Information Technology (BMIT) Research Group,
School of Information Technologies, University of Sydney, Sydney,
NSW, Australia
e-mail: tom.cai@sydney.edu.au

Pol Cirujeda
Department of Information and Communication Technologies,
Universitat Pompeu Fabra, Barcelona, Spain
e-mail: pol.cirujeda@upf.edu

Adrien Depeursinge
University of Applied Sciences Western Switzerland (HES-SO),
Sierre, Switzerland
e-mail: adrien.depeursinge@hevs.ch

Michel Desvignes
GIPSA-Lab, CNRS UMR 5216, Grenoble-INP, Université Joseph Fourier,
Saint Martin d'Hères, France
Université Stendhal, Saint Martin d'Hères, France
e-mail: michel.desvignes@gipsa-lab.grenoble-inp.fr

Ivan Eggel
Institute for Information Systems, University of Applied Sciences
Western Switzerland (HES–SO Valais), Sierre, Switzerland
e-mail: ivan.eggel@hevs.ch

Olof Enqvist
Department of Signals and Systems, Chalmers University of Technology,
Gothenburg, Sweden
e-mail: olof.enqvist@chalmers.se

Frida Fejne
Department of Signals and Systems, Chalmers University of Technology,
Gothenburg, Sweden
e-mail: fejne@chalmers.se

Antonio Foncubierta-Rodríguez
Computer Vision Laboratory, Swiss Federal Institute of Technology (ETH) Zurich,
Zurich, Switzerland
e-mail: antonio.foncubierta@vision.ee.ethz.ch

Johan Fredriksson
Centre for Mathematical Sciences, Lund University, Lund, Sweden
e-mail: johanf@maths.lth.se

Orcun Goksel
Computer Vision Laboratory, Swiss Federal Institute of Technology (ETH) Zurich,
Zurich, Switzerland
e-mail: ogoksel@ethz.ch

Katharina Grünberg
University of Heidelberg, Heidelberg, Germany
e-mail: katharina.gruenberg@med.uni-heidelberg.de

Allan Hanbury
TU Wien, Institute of Software Technology and Interactive Systems,
Vienna, Austria
e-mail: allan.hanbury@tuwien.ac.at

András Jakab
Medical University of Vienna, Vienna, Austria
e-mail: andras.jakab@meduniwien.ac.at

Oscar Jimenez-del-Toro
Institute of Information Systems, University of Applied Sciences
Western Switzerland Sierre (HES-SO), Sierre, Switzerland
e-mail: oscar.jimenez@hevs.ch

Leo Joskowicz
The Rachel and Selim Benin School of Computer Science and Engineering,
The Hebrew University of Jerusalem, Jerusalem, Israel
e-mail: leo.josko@mail.huji.ac.il

Fredrik Kahl
Department of Signals and Systems, Chalmers University of Technology,
Gothenburg, Sweden
Centre for Mathematical Sciences, Lund University, Lund, Sweden
e-mail: fredrik.kahl@chalmers.se

Razmig Kéchichian
CREATIS, CNRS UMR5220, Inserm U1044, INSA-Lyon,
Université de Lyon, Lyon, France
Université Claude Bernard Lyon 1, Lyon, France
e-mail: razmig.kechichian@creatis.insa-lyon.fr

Markus Krenn
Medical University of Vienna, Vienna, Austria
e-mail: markus.krenn@meduniwien.ac.at

Matilda Landgren
Centre for Mathematical Sciences, Lund University, Lund, Sweden
e-mail: matilda@maths.lth.se

Georg Langs
Medical University of Vienna, Vienna, Austria
e-mail: georg.langs@meduniwien.ac.at

Viktor Larsson
Centre for Mathematical Sciences, Lund University, Lund, Sweden
e-mail: viktorl@maths.lth.se

Henning Müller
Institute for Information Systems, University of Applied Sciences
Western Switzerland (HES–SO Valais), Sierre, Switzerland
University Hospitals and University of Geneva, Geneva, Switzerland
e-mail: henning.mueller@hevs.ch

Tomàs Salas Fernandez
Agencia D'Informació, Avaluació I Qualitat En Salut, Catalonia, Spain
e-mail: tomas.salas@gencat.cat

Roger Schaer
Institute for Information Systems, University of Applied Sciences
Western Switzerland (HES–SO Valais), Sierre, Switzerland
e-mail: roger.schaer@hevs.ch

Örjan Smedby
Center for Medical Image Science and Visualization (CMIV),
Linköping University, Linköping, Sweden
Department of Radiology and Department of Medical and Health Sciences,
Linköping University, Linköping, Sweden
School of Technology and Health (STH), KTH Royal Institute of Technology,
Stockholm, Sweden
e-mail: orjan.smedby@sth.kth.se

Yang Song
Biomedical and Multimedia Information Technology (BMIT)
Research Group, School of Information Technologies, University of Sydney,
Sydney, NSW, Australia
e-mail: yang.song@sydney.edu.au

Assaf B. Spanier
The Rachel and Selim Benin School of Computer Science and Engineering,
The Hebrew University of Jerusalem, Jerusalem, Israel
e-mail: assaf.spanier@mail.huji.ac.il

Johannes Ulén
Department of Signals and Systems, Chalmers University of Technology,
Gothenburg, Sweden
e-mail: ulen@maths.lth.se

Sébastien Valette
CREATIS, CNRS UMR5220, Inserm U1044, INSA-Lyon,
Université de Lyon, Lyon, France
Université Claude Bernard Lyon 1, Lyon, France
e-mail: sebastien.valette@creatis.insa-lyon.fr

Chunliang Wang
Center for Medical Image Science and Visualization (CMIV),
Linköping University, Linköping, Sweden
Department of Radiology and Department of Medical and Health Sciences,
Linköping University, Linköping, Sweden
School of Technology and Health (STH), KTH Royal Institute of Technology,
Stockholm, Sweden
e-mail: chunliang.wang@liu.se

Marc-André Weber
University of Heidelberg, Heidelberg, Germany
e-mail: marcandre.weber@med.uni-heidelberg.de

Marianne Winterstein
University of Heidelberg, Heidelberg, Germany
e-mail: marianne.winterstein@med.uni-heidelberg.de

Fan Zhang
Biomedical and Multimedia Information Technology (BMIT) Research Group,
School of Information Technologies, University of Sydney, Sydney,
NSW, Australia
e-mail: fzha8048@uni.sydney.edu.au

Acronyms

API	Application programming interface
BoVW	Bag of Visual Words
bpref	Binary preference
CAD	Computer-aided diagnosis
CECT	Contrast-enhanced CT
CLEF	Conference and Labs of the Evaluation Forum
CT	Computed tomography
Ctce	Contrast-enhanced computed tomography image
CVT	Centroidal Voronoi tessellation
DICOM	Digital Imaging and Communications in Medicine
EM	Expectation–maximization
EU	European Union
GM-MAP	Geometric mean average precision
HU	Hounsfield unit
IDF	Inverse document frequency
IRB	Internal review board
ISBI	International Symposium on Biomedical Imaging
k-NN	k-nearest neighbour
MAP	Mean average precision
MEC	Medical ethics committee
MR	Magnetic resonance
MRI	Magnetic resonance imaging
MRT1	Magnetic resonance T1-weighted image
MRT1cefs	Contrast-enhanced fat-saturated magnetic resonance T1-weighted image
MRT2	Magnetic resonance T2-weighted image
NIfTI	Neuroimaging Informatics Technology Initiative
NMI	Normalized mutual information
OS	Operating system
P10	Precision after 10 cases retrieved

P30	Precision after 30 cases retrieved
PACS	Picture archiving and communication systems
PCA	Principal component analysis
pLSA	Probabilistic Latent Semantic Analysis
QC	Quality control
RadLex	Radiology Lexicon
RANSAC	Random sample consensus
ROI	Region of interest
SIFT	Scale-invariant feature transform
SIMPLE	Selective and iterative method for performance level estimation
SURF	Speeded Up Robust Features
TF	Term frequency
TREC	Text Retrieval Conference
URL	Uniform resource locator
VISCERAL	Visual Concept Extraction Challenge in Radiology
VM	Virtual machine

Part I
Evaluation-as-a-Service

Chapter 1
VISCERAL: Evaluation-as-a-Service for Medical Imaging

Allan Hanbury and Henning Müller

Abstract Systematic evaluation has had a strong impact on many data analysis domains, for example, TREC and CLEF in information retrieval, ImageCLEF in image retrieval, and many challenges in conferences such as MICCAI for medical imaging and ICPR for pattern recognition. With Kaggle, a platform for machine learning challenges has also had a significant success in crowdsourcing solutions. This shows the importance to systematically evaluate algorithms and that the impact is far larger than simply evaluating a single system. Many of these challenges also showed the limits of the commonly used paradigm to prepare a data collection and tasks, distribute these and then evaluate the participants' submissions. Extremely large datasets are cumbersome to download, while shipping hard disks containing the data becomes impractical. Confidential data can often not be shared, for example medical data, and also data from company repositories. Real-time data will never be available via static data collections as the data change over time and data preparation often takes much time. The Evaluation-as-a-Service (EaaS) paradigm tries to find solutions for many of these problems and has been applied in the VISCERAL project. In EaaS, the data are not moved but remain on a central infrastructure. In the case of VISCERAL, all data were made available in a cloud environment. Participants were provided with virtual machines on which to install their algorithms. Only a small part of the data, the training data, was visible to participants. The major part of the data, the test data, was only accessible to the organizers who ran the algorithms in the participants' virtual machines on the test data to obtain impartial performance measures.

A. Hanbury (✉)
TU Wien, Institute of Software Technology and Interactive Systems,
Favoritenstraße 9-11/188, 1040 Vienna, Austria
e-mail: allan.hanbury@tuwien.ac.at

H. Müller
Information Systems Institute, HES-SO Valais,
Rue du Technopole 3, 3960 Sierre, Switzerland
e-mail: henning.mueller@hevs.ch

© The Author(s) 2017
A. Hanbury et al. (eds.), *Cloud-Based Benchmarking*
of Medical Image Analysis, DOI 10.1007/978-3-319-49644-3_1

3

1.1 Introduction

Scientific progress can usually be measured via clear and systematic experiments (Lord Kelvin: "If you can not measure it, you can not improve it."). In the past, scientific benchmarks, such as TREC (Text REtrieval Conference) and CLEF (Conference and Labs of the Evaluation Forum), have given a platform for such scientific comparisons and have had a significant impact [15, 17, 18]. Commercial platforms such as Kaggle[1] have also shown that there is a market for a comparison of techniques based on real problems that companies can propose.

Much data are available and can potentially be exploited for generating new knowledge based on data, including notably medical imaging, where extremely large amounts have been produced for many years [1]. Still, constraints are often that data need to be manually anonymized or can only be used in restricted settings, which does not work well for very large datasets.

Several of the problems encountered in traditional benchmarking that often relies on the paradigm of creating a dataset and sending it to participants can be summarized in the following points:

- *very large* datasets can only be distributed with very much effort, usually by sending hard disks through the post;
- *confidential* data are extremely hard to distribute, and they can usually only be used in a closed environment, in a hospital or inside the company firewalls;
- *quickly changing* datasets cannot be used for benchmarking if it is necessary to package the data and send them around.

To answer these problems and challenges, the VISCERAL project proposed a change in the way that benchmarking has been organized by proposing to keep the data in a central space and move the algorithms to the data [3, 10].

Other benchmarks equally realized these difficulties in running benchmarks and came up with a variety of propositions for running benchmarks without fixed data packages that are distributed. These ideas were discussed in a workshop organized around this topic and named Evaluation-as-a-Service (EaaS) [6]. Based on the discussions at the workshop, a detailed White Paper was written [4], which outlines the roles involved in this process and also the benefits that researchers, funding organizations and companies can gain from such a shift in scientific evaluations.

This chapter highlights the role of VISCERAL in the EaaS area, in which the benchmarks were organized and how the benchmarks helped advance this field and gain concrete experience with running scientific evaluations in the cloud.

---

[1] http://www.kaggle.com.

1.2 VISCERAL Benchmarks

The VISCERAL project organized a series of medical imaging Benchmarks described below:

1.2.1 Anatomy Benchmarks

A set of medical imaging data in which organs are manually annotated is provided to the participants. The data contain segmentations of several different anatomical structures and positions of landmarks in different image modalities, e.g. CT and MRI. Participants in the Anatomy Benchmarks have the task of submitting software that automatically segments the organs for which manual segmentations are provided, or detecting the locations of the landmarks. After submission, this software is tested on images which are inaccessible to the participants. Three rounds of the Anatomy Benchmark have been organized, and this Benchmark is continuing beyond the end of the VISCERAL project. These benchmarks are described in more detail in Chap. 7. In Chaps. 9–12 are reports of some participants in the Anatomy Benchmarks.

1.2.2 Detection Benchmark

A set of medical imaging data that contains various lesions manually annotated in anatomical regions such as the bones, liver, brain, lung or lymph nodes is distributed to the participants. Participants in the Detection Benchmark have the task of submitting software that will automatically detect these lesions. The software is tested on detecting lesions on images that the participants have not seen. The Benchmark data and ground truth continue to be available beyond the end of the VISCERAL project as the Detection2 Benchmark. As this was the most challenging benchmark that was organized, no solutions were submitted. There is therefore no chapter on this benchmark included, although the data and ground truth continue to be available.

1.2.3 Retrieval Benchmark

One of the challenges of medical information retrieval is similar case retrieval in the medical domain based on multimodal data, where cases refer to data about specific patients (used in an anonymized form), such as medical records, radiology images and radiology reports, or to cases described in the literature or teaching files. The Retrieval Benchmark simulates the following scenario: a medical professional is assessing a query case in a clinical setting, e.g. a CT volume, and is searching for cases that are relevant in this assessment. The participants in the Benchmark have the task of developing software that finds clinically relevant (related or useful for differential diagnosis) cases given a query case (imaging data only or imaging and text data), but not necessarily the final diagnosis. The Benchmark data and relevance assessments continue to be available beyond the end of the VISCERAL project as the Retrieval2 Benchmark. This benchmark is described in more detail in Chap. 8, and Chapters 13 and 14 give reports of two of the participants in the Retrieval Benchmark.

1.3 Evaluation-as-a-Service in VISCERAL

Evaluation-as-a-Service is an approach to the evaluation of data science algorithms, in which the data remain centrally stored, and participants are given access to these data in some controlled way.

The access to the data can be provided through various mechanisms, including an API to access the data, or virtual machines on which to install and run the processing algorithms. Mechanisms to protect sensitive data can also be implemented, such as running the virtual machines in sandboxed mode (all access out of the virtual machine is blocked) while the sensitive data are being processed, and destroying the virtual machine after extracting the results to ensure that no sensitive data remains in a virtual machine [13]. An overview of the use of Evaluation-as-a-Service is given in [4, 6].

We now give two examples of Evaluation-as-a-Service in use, illustrating the different types of data for which EaaS is useful. In the TREC Microblog task [11], search on Twitter was evaluated. As it is not permitted to redistribute tweets, an API (application programming interface) was created, allowing access to the tweets stored centrally. In the CLEF NewsREEL task [5], news recommender systems were evaluated. In this case, an online news recommender service sent requests for recommendations in real time based on actual requests from users, and the results were evaluated based on the clicks of the recommendations by the users of the online recommender service. As this was real-time data from actual users of a system, a platform, the Open Recommendation Platform [2], was developed to facilitate the communication between the news recommender portal and the task participants.

In the VISCERAL project, we were dealing with sensitive medical data. Even though the data had been anonymized by removing potentially personal metadata and blurring the facial regions of the images, it was not possible to guarantee that the anonymization tools had completely anonymized the images. We were therefore required to keep a large proportion of images, the test set, inaccessible to participants. Training images were available to participants as they had undergone a more thorough control of the anonymization effectiveness. The EaaS approach allowed this to be done in a straightforward way.

The training and test data are stored in the cloud in two separate storage containers. When each participant registers, he/she is provided with a virtual machine on the

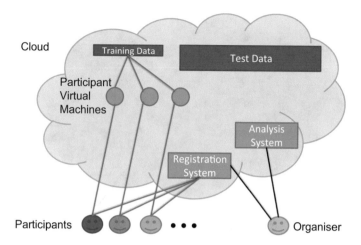

Fig. 1.1 Training Phase. The participants register, and each get their own virtual machine in the cloud, linked to a training dataset of the same structure as the test data. The software for carrying out the competition objectives is placed in the virtual machines by the participants. The test data are kept inaccessible to participants

cloud that has access to the training data container, as illustrated in Fig. 1.1. During the *Training Phase*, the participant should install the software that carries out the benchmark task on the virtual machine, following the specifications provided, and can train algorithms and experiment using the training data as necessary. Once the participant is satisfied with the performance of the installed software, the virtual machine is submitted to the organizers. Once a virtual machine is submitted, the participant loses access to it, and the *Test Phase* begins. The organizers link the submitted virtual machine to the test data, as shown in Fig. 1.2, run the submitted software on the test data and calculate metrics showing how well the submitted software performs.

For the initial VISCERAL benchmarks, the organizers set a deadline by which all virtual machines must be submitted. The values of the performance metrics were then sent to participants by email. This meant that a participant had only a single possibility to get the results of their computation on the test data. For the final round of the Anatomy Benchmark (Anatomy3), a continuous evaluation approach was adopted. Participants have the possibility to submit their virtual machine multiple times for the assessment of the software on the test set (there is a limit on how often this can be done to avoid "training on the test set"). The evaluation on the test set is carried out automatically, and participants can view the results on their personal results page. Participants can also choose to make results public on the global leaderboard.

Chapter 2 presents a detailed description of the VISCERAL cloud environment.

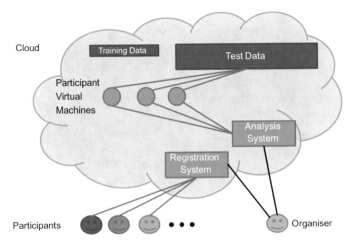

Fig. 1.2 Test Phase. On the Benchmark deadline, the organizer takes over the virtual machines containing the software written by the participants, links them to the test dataset, performs the calculations and evaluates the results

1.4 Main Outcomes of VISCERAL

As a result of running the Benchmarks, the VISCERAL project generated data and software that will continue to be useful to the medical imaging community. The first major data outcomes are manually annotated MR and CT images, which we refer to as the *Gold Corpus*. The use of the EaaS paradigm also gave the possibility to compute a *Silver Corpus* by fusing the results of the participant submissions. One of the challenges in creating datasets for use in medical imaging benchmarks is obtaining permission to use the image data for this purpose. In order to provide guidelines for researchers intending to obtain such permission, we present an overview of the processes necessary at the three institutes that provided data for the VISCERAL Benchmarks in Chap. 3. All data created during the VISCERAL project are described in detail in Chap. 5. Finally, particular attention was paid to ensuring that the metrics comparing segmentations were correctly calculated, leading to the release of new open source software for efficient metric calculation.

1.4.1 Gold Corpus

The VISCERAL project produced a large corpus of manually annotated radiology images, called the Gold Corpus. An innovative manual annotation coordination system was created, based on the idea of tickets, to ensure that the manual annotation was carried out as efficiently as possible. The Gold Corpus was subjected to an extensive quality control process and is therefore small but of high quality. Annotation

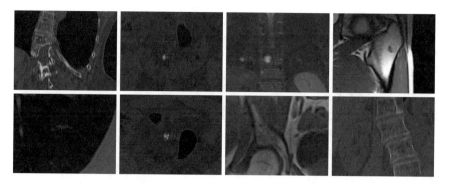

Fig. 1.3 Examples of lesion annotations

in VISCERAL served as the basis for all three Benchmarks. For each Benchmark, training data were distributed to the participants and testing data were kept for the evaluation.

For the Anatomy Benchmark series [8], volumes from 120 patients were manually segmented by the end of VISCERAL by radiologists, where the radiologists trace out the extent of each organ. The following organs were manually segmented: left/right kidney, spleen, liver, left/right lung, urinary bladder, rectus abdominis muscle, 1st lumbar vertebra, pancreas, left/right psoas major muscle, gallbladder, sternum, aorta, trachea and left/right adrenal gland. The radiologists also manually marked landmarks in the volumes, where the landmarks include lateral end of clavicula, crista iliaca, symphysis below, trochanter major, trochanter minor, tip of aortic arch, trachea bifurcation, aortic bifurcation and crista iliaca.

For the Detection Benchmark, overall 1,609 lesions were manually annotated in 100 volumes of two different modalities, in five different anatomical regions selected by radiologists: brain, lung, liver, bones and lymph nodes. Examples of the manual annotation of lesions are shown in Fig. 1.3.

For the Retrieval Benchmark [7], more than 10,000 medical image volumes were collected, from which about 2,000 were selected for the Benchmark. In addition, terms describing pathologies and anatomical regions were extracted from the corresponding radiology reports.

Detailed descriptions of the methods used in creating the Gold Corpus are described in Chap. 4.

1.4.2   Silver Corpus

In addition to the Gold Corpus of expert annotated imaging data described in the previous section, the use of the EaaS approach offered the possibility to generate a far larger Silver Corpus, which is annotated by the collective ensemble of participant algorithms. In other words, the Silver Corpus is created by fusing the outputs of all participant algorithms for each image (inspired by e.g. [14]). Even though this Silver Corpus annotation is less accurate than expert annotations, the fusion of participant algorithm results is more accurate than individual algorithms and offers a basis for large-scale learning. It was shown by experiments that the accuracy of a Silver Corpus annotation obtained by label fusion of participant algorithms is higher than the accuracy of individual participant annotations. Furthermore, this accuracy can be improved by injecting multi-atlas label fusion estimates of annotations based on the Gold Corpus-annotated dataset.

In effect, the Silver Corpus is large and diverse, but not of the same annotation quality as the Gold Corpus. The final Silver Corpus of VISCERAL Anatomy Benchmarks contains 264 volumes of four modalities (CT, CTce, MRT1 and MRT1cefs), containing 4193 organ segmentations and 9516 landmark annotations. Techniques for the creation of the Silver Corpus are described in [9].

1.4.3 Evaluation Metric Calculation Software

In order to evaluate the segmentations generated by the participants, it is necessary to compare them objectively to the manually created ground truth. There are many ways in which the similarity between two segmentations can be measured, and at least 22 metrics have each been used in more than one paper in the medical segmentation literature. We implemented these 22 metrics in the EvaluateSegmentation software [16], which is available as open source on GitHub,[2] and can read all image formats (2D and 3D) supported by the ITK Toolkit. The software is specifically optimized to be efficient and scalable, and hence can be used to compare segmentations on full body volumes. Chapter 6 goes beyond [16] by discussing the extension to fuzzy metrics and how well rankings based on similarity to the ground truth of organ segmentations by various metrics correlate with rankings of these segmentations by human experts.

1.5 Experience with EaaS in VISCERAL

Based on the examples given, there are several experiences to be gained from EaaS in general and VISCERAL more particularly. Some of the experiences, particularly in the medical domain, are also discussed in [12].

Initially, the idea to run an evaluation in the cloud was seen by the medical imaging community with some skepticism. Several persons mentioned that they would not participate if they cannot see the data and there definitely was a feeling of control loss. It is definitely additional work to install the required environment on a new virtual machine in the cloud. Furthermore, VISCERAL provided only a limited set

---

[2]https://github.com/Visceral-Project/EvaluateSegmentation.

of operating systems under Linux and Windows. There were also concrete questions regarding hardware such as GPU (graphical processing units) that are widely used for deep learning but that were not available in Azure at the time and prevented a potential participant from participating. These techniques are now easily available, so such problems are often removed quickly with the fast pace in the development of cloud infrastructures. Several participants who did not participate mentioned that they did so because it was additional work to set up the software in the cloud.

Other challenges were regarding the feedback when the algorithm completely failed for a specific image or when the script crashed. We had a few such cases and provided assistance to participants to remove the errors, but this is obviously only possible if the number of participants is relatively small.

In this respect, the system also created more work for the organizers than simply making data available for download and receiving calculated results from participants. Once infrastructures that are easier to use and a skeleton for evaluations are available, this will also reduce the additional work. The CodaLab[3] software is one such system that makes running a challenge in the cloud much easier, and a deeper integration between cloud and executed algorithms could help even further.

On the positive side are several important aspects. First, the three problems mentioned above regarding very large datasets, confidential data and quickly changing data are solved with the given approach. It is also important that all participants take part under the same conditions, so that there is no advantage with a fast Internet connection where data download takes minutes and not days. All participants also had the same environment, hence the same computing power, and there was no difference between computing resources available to participants, also removing a bias. The fact that all participating groups were compared based on the same infrastructure also allowed to compare run-time and thus efficiency of algorithms, which is impossible to compare otherwise. In terms of reproducibility, the system is extremely good as no one can optimize the techniques based on the test data.

The fact that the executables of all participants were available also allowed the creation of the Silver Corpus on new, non-annotated data, done by running all submitted algorithms on the new data and then performing a label fusion. This has shown to deliver much better results than even the best submitted algorithm. Availability of executables can also be used to run the code on new data that has become available or on modified data when errors were detected, something that did happen in VISCERAL.

The cloud-based evaluation workshop [12] also showed that there are several ongoing developments that will make the creation of such challenges and use of code much easier. Docker is, for example, much lighter than virtual machines, and submitting Docker containers can be both faster and reduce the amount of work necessary to create the container for participants. Code sharing among participants might also be supported in a more straightforward way, so participants can combine components of other research groups with their own components to optimize results systematically.

---

[3]https://github.com/codalab/.

1.6 Conclusion

The VISCERAL project made a number of useful contributions not only to the medical imaging field, but also to the organization of data science evaluations in general through advancing the Evaluation-as-a-Service approach. The techniques developed and lessons learned will be useful for the evaluation in machine learning, information retrieval, data mining and related areas, allowing the evaluation tasks to be done on huge, non-distributable, private or real-time data. This should not only allow the evaluation tasks to become more realistic and closer to practice, but should also increase the level of reproducibility of the experimental results.

In the area of medical imaging, the VISCERAL project contributed large datasets of annotated CT and MRI images. The annotations have been done by qualified radiologists in the creation of the Gold Corpus, but a form of crowdsourcing based on participant submissions allowed the much larger Silver Corpus to be built. Furthermore, a thorough analysis of metrics used in the evaluation of image segmentation was contributed, along with an efficient and scalable implementation of the calculation of these metrics.

Acknowledgements The research leading to these results has received funding from the European Union Seventh Framework Programme (FP7/2007-2013) under grant agreement 318068 (VISCERAL).

References

1. Riding the wave: how Europe can gain from the rising tide of scientific data (2010) Submission to the European commission. http://cordis.europa.eu/fp7/ict/e-infrastructure/docs/hlg-sdi-report.pdf
2. Brodt T, Hopfgartner F (2014) Shedding light on a living lab: the CLEF NEWSREEL open recommendation platform. In: IIiX'14: proceedings of information interaction in context conference. ACM, pp 223–226. http://dx.doi.org/10.1145/2637002.2637028
3. Hanbury A, Müller H, Langs G, Weber MA, Menze BH, Fernandez TS (2012) Bringing the algorithms to the data: cloud–based benchmarking for medical image analysis. In: Catarci T, Forner P, Hiemstra D, Peñas A, Santucci G (eds) CLEF 2012. LNCS, vol 7488. Springer, Heidelberg, pp 24–29. doi:10.1007/978-3-642-33247-0_3
4. Hanbury A, Müller H, Balog K, Brodt T, Cormack GV, Eggel I, Gollub T, Hopfgartner F, Kalpathy-Cramer J, Kando N, Krithara A, Lin J, Mercer S, Potthast M (2015) Evaluation-as-a-Service: overview and outlook. CoRR abs/1512.07454. http://arxiv.org/abs/1512.07454
5. Hopfgartner F, Kille B, Lommatzsch A, Plumbaum T, Brodt T, Heintz T (2014) Benchmarking news recommendations in a living lab. In: Kanoulas E, Lupu M, Clough P, Sanderson M, Hall M, Hanbury A, Toms E (eds) CLEF 2014. LNCS, vol 8685. Springer, Cham, pp 250–267. doi:10.1007/978-3-319-11382-1_21
6. Hopfgartner F, Hanbury A, Müller H, Kando N, Mercer S, Kalpathy-Cramer J, Potthast M, Gollub T, Krithara A, Lin J, Balog K, Eggel I (2015) Report on the Evaluation-as-a-Service (EaaS) expert workshop. SIGIR Forum 49(1):57–65
7. Jiménez-del-Toro O, Hanbury A, Langs G, Foncubierta-Rodríguez A, Müller H (2015) Overview of the VISCERAL retrieval benchmark 2015. In: Müller H, Jimenez del Toro O, Hanbury A, Langs G, Foncubierta Rodriguez A (eds) Multimodal retrieval in the medical

domain (MRMD) 2015. LNCS, vol 9059. Springer, Cham. doi:10.1007/978-3-319-24471-6_10

8. Jimenez-del-Toro O, Müller H, Krenn M, Gruenberg K, Taha AA, Winterstein M, Eggel I, Foncubierta-Rodríguez A, Goksel O, Jakab A, Kontokotsios G, Langs G, Menze B, Salas Fernandez T, Schaer R, Walleyo A, Weber MA, Dicente Cid Y, Gass T, Heinrich M, Jia F, Kahl F, Kechichian R, Mai D, Spanier AB, Vincent G, Wang C, Wyeth D, Hanbury A (2016) Cloud-based evaluation of anatomical structure segmentation and landmark detection algorithms: VISCERAL anatomy benchmarks. IEEE Trans Med Imaging

9. Krenn M, Dorfer M, Jiménez del Toro OA, Müller H, Menze B, Weber MA, Hanbury A, Langs G (2016) Creating a large-scale silver corpus from multiple algorithmic segmentations. In: Menze B, Langs G, Montillo A, Kelm M, Müller H, Zhang S, Cai W, Metaxas D (eds) MCV 2015. LNCS, vol 9601. Springer, Cham, pp 103–115. doi:10.1007/978-3-319-42016-5_10

10. Langs G, Hanbury A, Menze B, Müller H (2013) VISCERAL: towards large data in medical imaging — challenges and directions. In: Greenspan H, Müller H, Syeda-Mahmood T (eds) MCBR-CDS 2012. LNCS, vol 7723. Springer, Heidelberg, pp 92–98. doi:10.1007/978-3-642-36678-9_9

11. Lin J, Efron M (2013) Overview of the TREC-2013 microblog track. In: TREC'13: proceedings of the 22nd text retrieval conference, Gaithersburg, Maryland

12. Müller, Kalpathy-Cramer J, Hanbury A, Farahani K, Sergeev R, Paik JH, Klein A, Criminisi A, Trister A, Norman T, Kennedy D, Srinivasa G, Mamonov A, Preuss N (2016) Report on the cloud-based evaluation approaches workshop 2015. ACM SIGIR Forum 51(1):35–41

13. Potthast M, Gollub T, Rangel F, Rosso P, Stamatatos E, Stein B (2014) Improving the reproducibility of PAN's shared tasks: plagiarism detection, author identification, and author profiling. In: Kanoulas E, Lupu M, Clough P, Sanderson M, Hall M, Hanbury A, Toms E (eds) CLEF 2014. LNCS, vol 8685. Springer, Cham, pp 268–299. doi:10.1007/978-3-319-11382-1_22

14. Rebholz-Schuhmann D, Jimeno Yepes AJ, Van Mulligen EM, Kang N, Kors J, Milward D, Corbett P, Buyko E, Beisswanger E, Hahn U (2010) CALBC silver standard corpus. J Bioinform Comput Biol 8(1):163–179

15. Rowe BR, Wood DW, Link AN, Simoni DA (2010) Economic impact assessment of NIST text retrieval conference (TREC) program. Technical report project number 0211875, National Institute of Standards and Technology

16. Taha AA, Hanbury A (2015) Metrics for evaluating 3D medical image segmentation: analysis, selection, and tool. BMC Med Imaging 15(1):1–28

17. Thornley CV, Johnson AC, Smeaton AF, Lee H (2011) The scholarly impact of TRECVid (2003–2009). J Am Soc Info Sci Tech 62(4):613–627

18. Tsikrika T, Herrera AGS, Müller H (2011) Assessing the scholarly impact of ImageCLEF. In: Forner P, Gonzalo J, Kekäläinen J, Lalmas M, Rijke M (eds) CLEF 2011. LNCS, vol 6941. Springer, Heidelberg, pp 95–106. doi:10.1007/978-3-642-23708-9_12

Chapter 2
Using the Cloud as a Platform for Evaluation and Data Preparation

Ivan Eggel, Roger Schaer and Henning Müller

Abstract This chapter gives a brief overview of the VISCERAL Registration System that is used for all the VISCERAL Benchmarks and is released as open source on GitHub. The system can be accessed by both participants and administrators, reducing the direct participant–organizer interaction and handling the documentation available for each of the benchmarks organized by VISCERAL. Also, the upload of the VISCERAL usage and participation agreements is integrated, as well as the attribution of virtual machines that allow participation in the VISCERAL Benchmarks. In the second part, a summary of the various steps in the continuous evaluation chain mainly consisting of the submission, algorithm execution and storage as well as the evaluation of results is given. The final part consists of the cloud infrastructure detail, describing the process of defining requirements, selecting a cloud solution provider, setting up the infrastructure and running the benchmarks. This chapter concludes with a short experience report outlining the encountered challenges and lessons learned.

Source code is available at:
https://github.com/Visceral-Project/registration-system

I. Eggel (✉) · R. Schaer · H. Müller
Institute for Information Systems, University of Applied Sciences
Western Switzerland (HES–SO Valais), Sierre, Switzerland
e-mail: ivan.eggel@hevs.ch

R. Schaer
e-mail: roger.schaer@hevs.ch

H. Müller
University Hospitals and University of Geneva, Geneva, Switzerland
e-mail: henning.mueller@hevs.ch

2.1 Introduction

Over the past few years, medical imaging data have been steadily growing at a fast pace. In 2013, for instance, the Geneva University Hospitals produced around 300,000 images per day on average [8]. Working with increasingly big amounts of data has become difficult for researchers as the download of such big data would require a significant amount of time, especially in areas with slow Internet connections.

In the context of the VISCERAL Benchmarks where big data need to be shared with the participants, we decided to make use of a cloud infrastructure to host the data as well as to run the participants' code. On the one hand, this removes the necessity to download the data, and on the other hand, the participants are provided with equal-powered virtual machines in the cloud to run their code on, which makes the algorithms highly comparable in terms of performance. The evaluation infrastructure allows the Benchmarks to be carried out efficiently and effectively, along with a continuous evaluation allowing regular submission of virtual machines for evaluation. In order to register and administer the participants, but also to provide an interface between the participants and the cloud infrastructure, the VISCERAL Registration System has been developed.

2.2 VISCERAL Registration System

The VISCERAL project [5] has as a main goal to create an evaluation infrastructure for medical imaging tasks such as segmentation [7], lesion detection and retrieval [4]. An important part of the project was to create an innovative infrastructure for evaluating research algorithms on large image datasets and thus bringing the algorithms to the data instead of the data to the algorithms [2]. This is necessary when data grow large and image data have been identified as one of the main areas of large datasets [1].

In order for participants to have access to the cloud infrastructure provided by VISCERAL, participants have to register in the VISCERAL Registration System.[1] This system's purpose however is not restricted to registration of participants but also has the role of participant management system and additionally provides an interface between the participant and the cloud infrastructure, which hosts virtual machines and storage for the datasets. Figure 2.1 offers a simplified overview of the system for all steps needed from the registration process until the ability to view the participant's results. The approach of using such an integrated system for running benchmarks or competitions is highly recommended, significantly reducing administrative overhead regarding organizer–participant interaction as well as manual cloud configuration by the organizer, particularly if there is a large number of registering participants. Such

---

[1] http://visceral.eu:8080/register/Login.xhtml.

Fig. 2.1 Registration and subsequent processes from participant's and administrator's / system's point of view

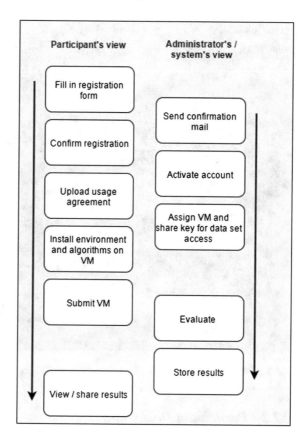

a system can also be used for continuous evaluation, allowing the participants to evaluate their algorithms at any time.

2.2.1 Registration

In the registration form, participants are asked to fill in their contact information including the affiliation and the benchmark in which they would like to participate. After receiving an email, the participants need to confirm their registration in order to obtain access to their personal dashboard. From there, the VISCERAL end-user agreement needs to be downloaded, printed and signed. An upload function allows for an upload of a scanned copy of the end-user agreement which, upon approval by the organizer, grants access to the VISCERAL dataset and the login credentials for a virtual machine (VM) in the cloud.

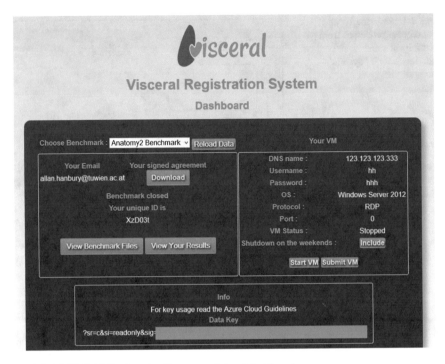

Fig. 2.2 VISCERAL Registration System participant dashboard

2.2.2 Participant Dashboard

After a successful registration and verification process, the participants are given an extended view on their dashboard as shown in Fig. 2.2, mainly providing:

- **Access details for VM and dataset** A VM, depending on the operating system (OS) platform, is accessed with a specific protocol (SSH for Linux, RemoteDesktop for Windows) and the credentials. In order for the participants to access the dataset (read-only), a specific data key is provided.
- **Start/stop VM** Starting/stopping a VM from the dashboard was implemented due to the fact that running a VM in the cloud causes financial costs, especially if it is never turned off during an extended period of time. Like this, participants who are not executing code are able to turn off their machines without requiring a direct access to the cloud management system. It needs to be mentioned that during the first benchmark, several participants left their VMs active over many weeks without executing code, resulting in unnecessary costs. In order to partially resolve this problem, an automatic shutdown of all VMs was introduced, scheduled every Friday evening, unless a participant excludes their VM from this shutdown using the option in the dashboard.

- **Download of benchmark files** Benchmark files are files that provide additional information on a specific benchmark. This can represent information such as URLs of files in the dataset that can be accessed from a VM, cloud usage guidelines or a data handling tutorial. The goal of these files is to give useful and clear information to the participant on how to use the system, the cloud and the dataset, significantly reducing email exchange between the participant and organizer by preventing simple recurring questions.
- **Submit VM** After the installation of necessary libraries and algorithms inside the provided VM, the participant can submit their VM from their dashboard in order for the algorithm to be evaluated for its performance. Exact instructions on how to submit a VM and on what exactly must be provided in the VM are provided in the form of a benchmark file.
- **View results** As soon as the evaluation has completed, the participant is able to view the results in the dashboard by modality, body region, organ and configuration. Results explicitly granted to be published by participants are shown in the publicly visible leaderboard.

2.2.3   Management of Participants

System administrators have access to the administration dashboard (Fig. 2.3) that displays all registered users relative to a selected Benchmark. In order to facilitate the participant management, different colours highlight the participant's status. A grey background is used to indicate that a participant has registered but has not yet

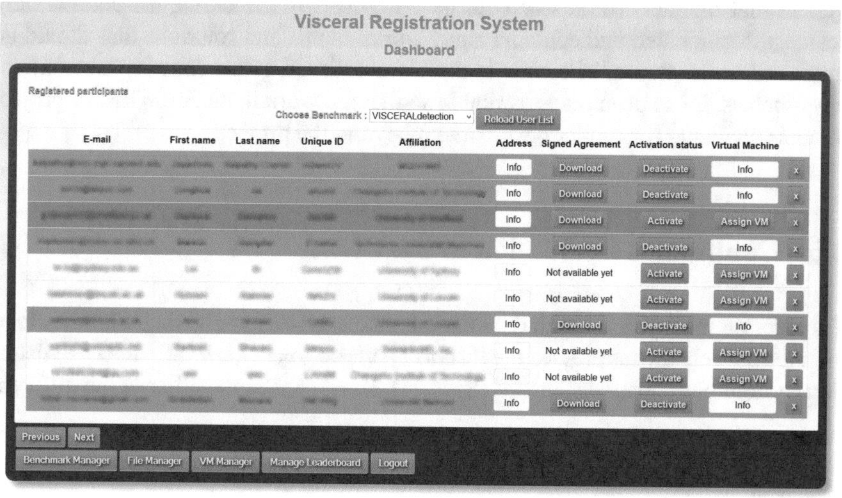

Fig. 2.3 VISCERAL Registration System administrator dashboard

uploaded the VISCERAL end-user agreement. A blue background suggests that a participant is waiting for administrator verification and account activation after the upload of the VISCERAL end-user agreement. A yellow background is shown upon activation of the participant account, meaning that the participant is ready to be assigned a VM, whereas a green background indicates that all previous steps have been successfully carried out. It is also possible for an administrator to create new benchmarks as well as to manage existing ones (Benchmark Manager), e.g. by editing starting and ending dates. In order to administer the files with additional information for each benchmark (benchmark files, Sect. 2.2.2), the File Manager is used. Besides that, administrators are also able to access and edit the information for the VM of each participant by consulting the VM Manager. Various tasks relative to the management of VMs, such as starting/stopping a VM and monitoring the current status of all VMs, are done in this place. The Leaderboard Manager is used for viewing/editing results for a specific organ that participants explicitly made available for the public (as described in Sect. 2.2.2).

2.2.4   Open Source Software Release

The registration system was built with the Java EE[2] platform and Git[3] was used for the software management. On GitHub, the project source is publicly available[4] under GNU General Public License for anyone to review and extend as they wish. Committing changes on the original codebase is not possible and requires the relevant privileges to be given. The aim in writing this code was to demonstrate the concept of cloud-based evaluation through having a working registration and administration system for the benchmarks. Due to this being the first version of the registration system that interacts so closely with the Microsoft Azure cloud, the code is only scarcely documented and contains many workarounds and solutions that should be improved in the future. The code is therefore not well suited for easy installation; nevertheless, it has been made available so that the work in the VISCERAL project remains available for further development beyond the project.

2.3   Continuous Evaluation in the Cloud

This section mainly deals with the internals of the system interacting with the cloud after the participant has pressed the Submit VM button in the VISCERAL Registration System participant dashboard (Sect. 2.2.2). A brief explanation of the different

---

[2]Java Platform, Enterprise Edition: http://www.oracle.com/technetwork/java/javaee/overview/index.html.

[3]https://git-scm.com/.

[4]https://github.com/Visceral-Project/registration-system.

steps in the partly automated approach for the evaluation of segmentations on the test set generated by software submitted by participants is given. The high level of automation permits participants to submit their software multiple times to obtain results during a benchmark.

2.3.1 Submission

Before submitting a VM, the participant is asked to provide an executable in a specific directory, which takes a set of parameters defined by the organizer. The participant has to make sure that the executable properly calls their algorithms and is able to work with data in the cloud. In order to do so, participants have to accurately follow the instructions provided in the benchmark files. Clearer instructions generally mean that fewer problems occur when running the executable during the evaluation, resulting in less administrative overhead on the organizers' side.

2.3.2 Isolation of the VM

In order to prevent the participants from accessing and manipulating the VM after the submission, i.e. during the test phase, a Web service is called from the VISCERAL Registration System as soon as a participant submits the VM. This Web service isolates the VM by creating a firewall rule in the cloud, blocking all remote access from outside the cloud. A second rule is created to explicitly allow certain ranges of IP addresses for the organizers. These rules are removed after the test phase has terminated.

2.3.3 Initial Test

Letting participants run their own code on a VM can be error-prone, as the first benchmark organized has shown. Submitted code often contains bugs or unhandled exceptions that make the evaluation fail. In order to prevent such situations in a limited way, the system tests the participant's executable prior to the final evaluation. For this test, both a batch script and a list of URLs of the test set files are downloaded to the VM. The script calls the participant's executable for a single test volume and ensures the match between output files and those expected by the participant. In case the test fails, the VM is automatically shut down and returned to the participant in order to fix the faults present in their code.

2.3.4 Executing Algorithms and Saving the Results

After the initial test, the batch script is called in order to execute the participant's executable for every volume contained in the test set as well as for each of the allowed configurations. A temporary drive in the VM is used in order to store the output files. The batch scripts require to provide the test set URL list, the output directory, the participant ID and the benchmark as arguments.

In order to make the results public and persistent, after the generation of each output file they are automatically uploaded to the cloud storage account and removed from the VM's temporary drive in order to ensure sufficient storage space for subsequent files. The process of storing the output file to the cloud storage is performed with a secure Web service (HTTPS) connecting to the cloud provider's API. The files are stored in a folder dedicated to the participants' results inside the storage container.

2.3.5 Evaluation of Results

The results are evaluated using the EvaluateSegmentation[5] [6] software developed during the VISCERAL project. As soon as the output files are generated and stored in the cloud storage as described in Sect. 2.3.4, a script is called in order to evaluate and save the results in two steps:

- For each output file (segmentation), the EvaluateSegmentation tool is called in order to compare the segmentation with its corresponding ground truth. This results in an XML file with 20 evaluation metrics.
- After this, the XML file is parsed and the metrics are inserted into a database in which each dataset contains all information corresponding to a single metric value, e.g. metric id, participant id, volume, modality, and organ. These data are then displayed to the participant in the result dashboard or optionally in the leaderboard (Sect. 2.2.2).

2.4 Cloud-Based Evaluation Infrastructure

This section details the technical and administrative aspects of setting up a cloud-based evaluation infrastructure, such as analysing the requirements, choosing a cloud provider and estimating the costs. The basic concept consists of storing large amounts of data in the cloud and providing participants in benchmarks with virtual machines (VMs) where they can access these data, install software and test their algorithms for a given task (illustrated in Fig. 2.4).

---

[5]https://github.com/codalab/EvaluateSegmentation.

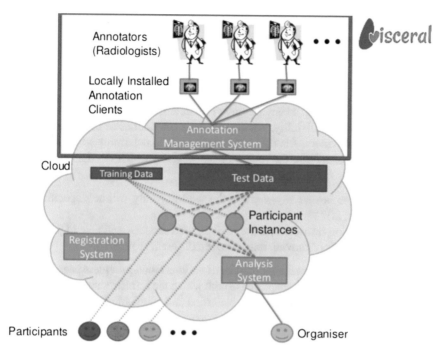

Fig. 2.4 Overview of the VISCERAL Cloud Framework. In the *upper* part (*red rectangle*), the process of data creation is described. Radiologists manually annotate images on locally installed clients and then submit their data to the annotation management system. From there, the training and testing sets are generated. Subsequently, participants who have registered and obtained a virtual machine can access their instance and optimize their algorithms and methods on the training data. Finally, the virtual machine is submitted by the participants, and the control is given to the organizer, who can then run the participant's executable on the testing set and perform the evaluation of the results while the participant has no access

2.4.1 Setting up a Cloud Environment

Selecting and configuring a cloud environment require the analysis of several points, which are detailed in this section. The analysis of requirements as well as the evaluation of costs and logistical aspects are investigated.

2.4.1.1 Requirements

Cloud-based solution providers offer many products, including:

- Data storage, both structured (database) and unstructured (files);
- Computation with virtual machines;
- Authentication and security mechanisms;
- Application-specific features:

– distributed computing (e.g. Hadoop[6]);
– high-performance computing;
– media services (e.g. video transcoding);
– monitoring tools;
– content caching.

The first step in setting up an environment is to determine which features are needed and to compare the availability, pricing and usage modalities of these features with different cloud providers. Another important step is to determine whether there are any restrictions concerning the region of the world in which the data and services are hosted. Sample questions include the following:

• Can the data be hosted anywhere in the world or only within a specific region (USA, Europe, ...)?
• If there is a region restriction, are all the required services available in this region?
• What are the costs of moving data between different regions?

Carefully reviewing the usage modalities of various cloud providers is an important step that can potentially impact the ease with which the infrastructure can be put into place. Once the required features are identified and a suitable provider is selected, the next step is planning the set-up of the environment.

2.4.1.2   Costs and Logistics

When planning the set-up of a cloud environment, it is important to evaluate the needs in terms of required resources, both to have a clear idea of the administrative workload (managing virtual machines, storage containers, access rights, etc.) and to estimate the costs of maintaining the infrastructure. All major cloud providers have cost-calculating tools, making it easier to make an accurate approximation of monthly costs. Depending on the provider, different components can add to the total cost:

• Storage

    – Data stored (usually billed as Gigabytes per month);
    – Incoming / outgoing data traffic (usually billed per Gigabyte, incoming traffic is typically free);
    – Storage requests (PUT/COPY/POST/LIST/GET HTTP requests);

• Virtual Machines

    – Running virtual machines (usually billed by the hour);
    – Virtual machine attached storage;
    – Data transfer to and from the virtual machines;
    – Additional IP addresses.

---

[6]http://hadoop.apache.org.

The costs also depend on the usage scenarios:

- Are data stored only for short periods and then removed, or do they need to be available for months or years?
- Are virtual machines required to be running 24/7 or are they used periodically for heavy computation and then turned off?
- Are Windows virtual machines required? (they are generally more expensive than Linux-based instances because of licensing costs).

Making cost projections for several months or a year can help in managing the resources more efficiently and making adjustments before the costs exceed expectations. Another aspect of the planning phase is to think about the resource management tasks involved. Any manual tasks can quickly become daunting when they need to be performed on a multitude of virtual machines. Properly configuring the base images used for future virtual machine instances can save much time and help in avoiding technical problems. Initial configuration tasks include the following:

- Setting sensible values for password expiration and complexity requirements;
- Disabling unscheduled reboots on automatic update installation;
- Configuring the system's firewall if any ports need to be accessible from the outside.

2.4.2 Setting up a Benchmark in the Cloud

Once the cloud provider is selected and the infrastructure requirements are defined, a workflow for an evaluation benchmark needs to be created. This workflow includes at least the following elements:

- Description of the different phases of the benchmark:
  - examples: dataset creation, training phase and test phase;
  - define what should happen in each phase and who is responsible for which task;
- Required security measures:
  - geographic location of the data and infrastructure;
  - access control for participants and administrators: time restrictions for accessing the data, user rights, etc;
  - create security protocols: firewall software, antivirus, end-user agreement;
- Creation of the required resources for the various phases:
  - storage containers for the data
    · different containers for the phases (training, test) are recommended. It makes locating and data management easier;
  - virtual machines for computation

· creation of preconfigured machine templates (images) is recommended; it allows avoiding additional manual configuration on each machine after creation;

· the variety of operating systems provided to the participants impacts the administrative workload involved in setting up the infrastructure; managing both Linux and Windows instances can make administrative tasks and automation more difficult, requiring at least two variants of all used scripts or tools;

• Definition of data exchange protocols between the participants and the cloud infrastructure:

– how can participants upload / download data to and from the cloud;
– Are there additional data needed for the benchmark located outside the cloud (registration system, documentation...)?

2.4.3 Cloud Set-Up for the VISCERAL Benchmarks

The VISCERAL project was hosted in the Microsoft Azure cloud. The usage of a public cloud platform such as Microsoft Azure enabled virtually unlimited scalability, in terms of both storage space and computation power. The Microsoft Azure platform provides a framework for the creation and management of virtual machines and data storage containers, among a large offer of services. The platform's Web management portal was used for the VISCERAL project to simplify the administrative tasks. A large amount of documentation and tools used for the different administrative tasks and technical aspects of the project are described on the Microsoft Azure Website. Provision and management of VMs, as well as data storage, were the main cloud services used during the project. In the following paragraphs, a brief description of these services is given.

2.4.3.1 Storing Datasets

Initially, the full dataset with both the medical data and the additional annotations created by expert radiologists was uploaded to a cloud storage container. Other cloud storage containers were then created in each benchmark to store the training and test datasets, participant output files and evaluations. Time-restricted read-only access keys were distributed securely to the participants for accessing the training datasets. Participants had no access to the test set and subsequent evaluation results. Over the course of the project, new images and their annotations were added to the storage containers when required.

2.4.3.2 Participant VMs

In order to run the VISCERAL benchmarks, the participants needed access to the stored data and computing instances to execute their algorithms. Virtual machines running on the Microsoft Azure cloud infrastructure were preconfigured to run these tasks. Different templates were configured for five operating systems including both Windows and Linux. A virtual machine was provided to each participant, allowing them to access the training dataset and upload their algorithms. Each VM has a temporary storage space where the participant output files are stored during the test phase. These temporary data are deleted each time the VM is shut down. All the participant VM instances have the same computing specifications and capabilities. Participants can remotely access their VMs during the training phase. Moreover, they can install all the tools and libraries needed to run their algorithms. At this stage, they can optimize their approaches with the available training set. Specification guidelines were written by the administrators for each benchmark on the usage and permissions applying to the VMs. Through the participant dashboard in the VISCERAL registration and management system, participants received the private access credentials for the their VM and had the option to start it or shut it down during the training phase. All the benchmark specifications and usage guidelines were also available in the dashboard.

2.4.4 Cloud Infrastructure Setup and Management Experience Report

The VISCERAL project organized the first series of benchmarks with a large-scale 3D radiology image dataset using an innovative cloud-based evaluation approach. Having the data stored centrally yields legal, administrative and practical solutions to organizing benchmarks with large datasets:

- The data can be allocated in a private storage container that complies with the legal requirements from the data providers (also HIPAA compliant—Health Insurance Portability and Accountability Act).
- Better control over the project costs, since a cloud platform is flexible enough to increase or reduce the number of VMs and storage containers according to the shifting challenge needs.
- The scalability and storage capacity of a cloud platform are virtually unlimited. This feature opens up the possibility to run benchmarks on big datasets with a high number of participants.
- Different access permissions to the data are defined by the organizers with the option to make some information inaccessible to the participants (e.g. test set).
- The submitted algorithms can be evaluated by the administrators without the intervention from the participants. This generates an objective evaluation of the execution and results.

2.4.4.1 Lessons Learned

In retrospective, the following steps were highlighted due to their favourable influence in the benchmark success:

- Planning must consider every component of the platform and how to seamlessly connect them when running the benchmarks. Some early decisions in the project can have a decisive effect in the long term of the evaluation process.
- Clear specifications are paramount and should be defined in great detail from the beginning. Both organizers and participants need to rely on these specifications throughout the project.
- Continuous assessment of the infrastructure needs to be based on the participant feedback. The updates coming from these assessments need to be well documented and transparent to the participants.

2.4.4.2 Current Challenges

Running benchmarks in the cloud is a significant paradigm shift [3] and requires an adaptation period, both from the benchmark organizers and from the participant perspective. It can be challenging to move away from the classic model of providing the data to the participants (i.e. downloading the datasets via traditional file transfer protocols such as FTP) and towards the new way of bringing the participants to the data (i.e. giving the participants data access through a virtual machine in the cloud). Outlined in this section are some pending challenges to consider for future benchmark organizers:

- **Narrow time frame for planning, setting up the infrastructure and running benchmarks**: Access and usage of a cloud platform requires a learning period for most of the participants. Strict timelines for isolated benchmarks can limit the number of participants that go through the process of registering, training their algorithms and submitting their VMs. Having a continuous cycle of benchmarks (e.g. annual events) might attract more participants to adapt their algorithms in the cloud and eventually submit the results for the benchmarks. This is not always possible because of the strict timelines to run the benchmarks and analyse the participants' results for a finite number of competitions.
- **Freedom to adapt the cloud platform**: Apart from data security and confidentiality considerations, using a public cloud environment can impact the level of customization available to administrators. The provided management tools need to be used "as is", and little to no possibilities exist to adapt them to more specific needs. Scheduled maintenance operations can also make the platform unavailable or cause disruptions in the benchmark workflow. A private cloud may provide a more flexible environment to develop an evaluation framework. On the other hand, a public cloud simplifies setting up and maintaining the backbone of the platform and theoretically allows for limitless scalability. Choosing the right cloud computing option depends on the initial objectives of the benchmark.

- **Some of the components of the VISCERAL infrastructure were implemented outside the Azure cloud platform**: This was mainly due to the limited time frame to set up the needed infrastructure for running and preparing the benchmarks in the cloud. Technical limitations, such as reduced Internet connection speed, as well as unfamiliarity of the users with the cloud environment were also hurdles in setting up the benchmarks. Having all the system components in the cloud would have allowed for a more streamlined benchmark organization process.
- **No uniform participant working environments**: Managing different operating systems and heterogeneous participant prototyping languages and tools increased the workload of setting up the infrastructure: compilation of evaluation tools for different platforms, handling OS differences in the automation process (Windows, Linux), VM maintenance, etc. Using a single family of OS could harmonize the infrastructure management tasks. However, this might result in less participation overall.

2.5 Conclusion

With a high number of participants in an evaluation benchmark, the administrative tasks for organizers represent a large amount of work. Using a system providing a high level of automation, the amount of work by organizers as well participants can be significantly reduced. In order to achieve this, the VISCERAL Registration System, which is a platform that provides participant management and an interface between participants and organizers as well as between participants and the cloud, was developed. Participants in the VISCERAL benchmarks have used this system not only to register for the various benchmarks but also to indirectly interact with the organizers and the cloud infrastructure. The main functionalities of the system included the handling of the registration process, the account activation, the management of end-user agreements, the assignment and the submission of the VMs as well as the evaluation and the storage / provision of results. The development of such a system helped us to greatly reduce the time spent on administrative tasks such as email exchange with participants and manual cloud interaction. Using a similar approach for running future competitions or benchmarks in the cloud can thus be highly recommended.

The use of a cloud-based infrastructure allowed straightforward scaling up of the VISCERAL benchmarks in terms of storage space and computation power (i.e. number of participants). Centralizing the data and providing standardized virtual machine instances to participants allowed us to streamline the management of the evaluation procedure. Certain crucial aspects that should be taken into consideration when setting up an Evaluation-as-a-Service platform were highlighted during the project, such as the importance of exhaustive planning and definition of clear specifications. Minimizing manual tasks and parts of the platform running outside the cloud infrastructure can help save large amounts of time, especially as the number of participants increases. Cloud-based evaluation platforms certainly represent the future and will become more used as researchers get familiar with this new paradigm.

Acknowledgements The research leading to these results has received funding from the European Union Seventh Framework Programme (FP7/2007-2013) under grant agreement 318068 (VIS-CERAL).

References

1. Riding the wave: how Europe can gain from the rising tide of scientific data (2010) Submission to the European Commission. http://cordis.europa.eu/fp7/ict/e-infrastructure/docs/hlg-sdi-report. pdf
2. Hanbury A, Müller H, Langs G, Weber MA, Menze BH, Fernandez TS (2012) Bringing the algorithms to the data: cloud-based benchmarking for medical image analysis. In: Catarci T, Forner P, Hiemstra D, Peñas A, Santucci G (eds) CLEF 2012. LNCS, vol 7488. Springer, Heidelberg, pp 24–29. doi:10.1007/978-3-642-33247-0_3
3. Hopfgartner F, Hanbury A, Müller H, Kando N, Mercer S, Kalpathy-Cramer J, Potthast M, Gollub T, Krithara A, Lin J, Balog K, Eggel I (2015) Report on the Evaluation-as-a-Service (EaaS) expert workshop. ACM SIGIR Forum 49(1):57–65
4. Jiménez–del–Toro OA, Hanbury A, Langs G, Foncubierta–Rodríguez A, Müller H (2015) Overview of the VISCERAL retrieval benchmark 2015. In: Müller H, Jimenez del Toro OA, Hanbury A, Langs G, Foncubierta Rodríguez A (eds) Multimodal retrieval in the medical domain. LNCS, vol 9059. Springer, Cham, pp 115–123. doi:10.1007/978-3-319-24471-6_10
5. Langs G, Hanbury A, Menze B, Müller H (2013) VISCERAL: towards large data in medical imaging — challenges and directions. In: Greenspan H, Müller H, Syeda-Mahmood T (eds) MCBR-CDS 2012. LNCS, vol 7723. Springer, Heidelberg, pp 92–98. doi:10.1007/978-3-642-36678-9_9
6. Taha AA, Hanbury A (2015) Metrics for evaluating 3D medical image segmentation: analysis, selection, and tool. BMC Med Imaging 15(1):
7. Jiménez del Toro OA, Goksel O, Menze B, Müller H, Langs G, Weber MA, Eggel I, Gruenberg K, Holzer M, Kotsios-Kontokotsios G, Krenn M, Schaer R, Taha AA, Winterstein M, Hanbury A (2014) VISCERAL—VISual Concept Extraction challenge in RAdioLogy: ISBI 2014 challenge organization. In: Goksel O (ed) Proceedings of the VISCERAL challenge at ISBI, Beijing, China, vol 1194 in CEUR workshop proceedings, pp 6–15
8. Widmer A, Schaer R, Markonis D, Müller H (2014) Gesture interaction for content-based medical image retrieval. In: ICMR'14 proceedings of international conference on multimedia retrieval. ACM, New York, p 503

Part II
VISCERAL Datasets

Chapter 3
Ethical and Privacy Aspects of Using Medical Image Data

Katharina Grünberg, Andras Jakab, Georg Langs, Tomàs Salas Fernandez, Marianne Winterstein, Marc-André Weber, Markus Krenn and Oscar Jimenez-del-Toro

Abstract This chapter describes the ethical and privacy aspects of using medical data in the context of the VISCERAL project. The project had as main goals the creation of a benchmark for organ segmentation, landmark detection, lesion detection and similar case retrieval. The availability of a large amount of imaging data was extremely important for the project goals, and thus, we present an analysis of the procedures that were followed for getting access to the data from IRB (internal review board) approval to data extraction and usage. This chapter details the requirements stated by medical ethics committees in three partner countries that supplied data. The exact procedure from request to data distribution is explained. The specific requirements of each data provider (each from a different country) are described in detail. The final data collection was made available in anonymized form in the Microsoft Azure cloud with the restriction of having it on servers that are located inside the European Union.

K. Grünberg · M. Winterstein · M.-A. Weber
University of Heidelberg, Heidelberg, Germany
e-mail: katharina.gruenberg@med.uni-heidelberg.de

A. Jakab · G. Langs · M. Krenn
Medical University of Vienna, Vienna, Austria

G. Langs
e-mail: georg.langs@meduniwien.ac.at

T. Salas Fernandez
Agencia D'Informció, Avaluació i Qualitat en Salut, Catalonia (GENCAT), Spain

O. Jimenez-del-Toro (✉)
University of Applied Sciences Western Switzerland (HES–SO), Sierre, Switzerland
e-mail: oscar.jimenez@hevs.ch

© The Author(s) 2017
A. Hanbury et al. (eds.), *Cloud-Based Benchmarking
of Medical Image Analysis*, DOI 10.1007/978-3-319-49644-3_3

3.1 Introduction

The VISCERAL project developed a cloud-based infrastructure for evaluation of
analysis and search tasks on large medical image data sets and organized benchmarks
to exploit and compare multiple state-of-the-art solutions designed for segmentation,
landmark localization and search [1, 2]. The main Benchmarks focused on automatic
identification, localization and segmentation of organs in imaging (Anatomy Benchmarks) [3]. Through VISCERAL, different computational algorithms are brought to
large medical imaging datasets to support the evaluation of novel tools for the clinical
diagnostic image assessment and workflow. VISCERAL resulted in two types of databases as an open resource: the Gold Corpus with expert manual annotations and the
Silver Corpus with data computed from benchmark participants' algorithms [4]. This
chapter describes the aspects related to ethics, privacy and the legal basis of the data
use, and how the project consortium dealt with them during the project. This chapter
gives an overview of the common aspects and highlights the aspects depending on

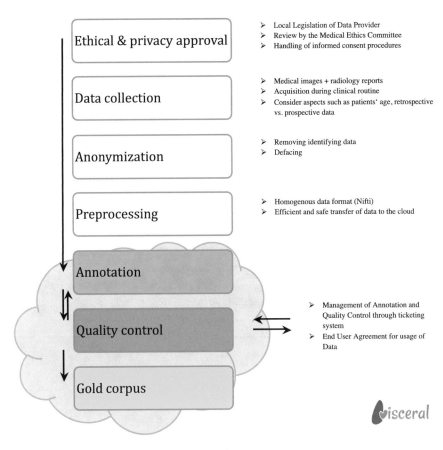

Fig. 3.1 An outline of the steps for data preparation

the country that provided the data. Figure 3.1 shows the data preparation outline to demonstrate the process from getting ethics approval to transferring the data to the cloud platform, where it is harmonized, e.g. transferred to the NIfTI (Neuroimaging Informatics Technology Initiative) format, annotated and quality controlled (see Chap. 4 for a detailed description of the latter steps).

3.2 Ethical and Privacy Aspects for Data Access

The data used in the project consisted of human medical imaging data and their corresponding meta-information. Therefore, its use was subject to specific regulations on both the European Union (EU) and national level that controlled the collection, use, distribution of human data and its inclusion in research studies. There were three data providers in the project:

1. Universitätsklinikum Heidelberg (UKL-HD), Germany
2. Agència d'Informació, Avaluació i Qualitat en Salut (GENCAT), Spain
3. Medizinische Universität Wien (MUW), Austria

Each data provider was responsible for handling the ethical, legal and privacy aspects relevant to the data provided by their group. This typically involves the following:

1. Review of the data collection plan by the local competent medical ethics committee (MEC) / institutional review board (IRB).
2. Handling of informed consent procedures.
3. Anonymization of the data prior to any use or distribution.

Relevant points from these procedures are addressed in more detail in the following sections.

3.2.1 Review by the Medical Ethics Committee

When applying for ethical approval from the competent local/national Ethics Committees, detailed information is provided regarding the following:

- The procedures that are used for the recruitment of participants (e.g. number of participants, inclusion/exclusion criteria, direct/indirect incentives for participation, and the risks and benefits for the participants).
- The nature of the material that will be collected (e.g. imaging data or additional structure data or free text reports).
- It must be explicitly stated if children or adults unable to give informed consent will be involved and, if so, justification for their participation must be provided.
- Detailed information on the informed consent procedures that are implemented.

Before the inclusion of data into the study, the review by the competent local MEC has to be concluded, and the study plan has to be approved by the MEC.

3.2.2 Handling of Informed Consent Procedures

Free informed consent by participants in a medical study is a prime aspect of the ethical considerations concerning medical research. The Declaration of Helsinki states that: *"The World Medical Association (WMA) has developed the Declaration of Helsinki as a statement of ethical principles for medical research involving human subjects, including research on identifiable human material and data"*, and *"After ensuring that the potential subject has understood the information, the physician or another appropriately qualified individual must then seek the potential subject's freely-given informed consent, preferably in writing."* [5]. More detailed discussions are given in [6, 7]. To fulfil the requirements of free informed consent, a participant has to have the right:

- to know that participation is voluntary;
- to ask questions and receive understandable answers before making a decision;
- to know the degree of risk and burden involved in participation;
- to know who will benefit from participation;
- to know the procedures that are implemented in the case of incidental findings;
- to receive assurance that appropriate insurance cover is in place;
- to withdraw themselves, their samples and data from the project at any time;
- to know how their biological samples and data are collected, protected during the project and destroyed at the end; and
- to know of any potential commercial exploitation of the research.

In the context of *retrospective studies* using data acquired prior to study start, and where the collection of informed consent is not feasible or possible, benefits and risks have to be weighted by the competent MEC. There is a discussion regarding research on biological material in the context of biobanks in Tassé et al. [8]. The authors note *"If it is not possible to recontact participants for reconsent, some guidelines allow for waived consent for the use of biological material, if certain conditions are met [9]. However, these conditions are not harmonized among international guidelines."* The authors conclude further *"As stated in the Declaration of Helsinki, ethical principles apply to 'medical research involving human subjects, including research on identifiable human material or identifiable data'. It follows that research using anonymised or anonymous data does not create an obligation to obtain informed consent, as the study does not involve identifiable individuals"*, taking [5, 10] into account. In [10] the relevant paragraphs emphasize the role of the local competent MEC in the decision of whether consent or reconsent is necessary if anonymized data are used:

- *"11. Under certain conditions, personal health information may be included in a database without consent, for example where this conforms with applicable national law that conforms to the requirements of this statement, or where ethical approval was given by a specifically appointed ethical review committee. In these exceptional cases, patients should be informed about the potential uses of their information, even if they have no right to object."*

- *"14. Approval from a specifically appointed ethical review committee must be obtained for all research using patient data, including for new research not envisaged at the time the data were collected. An important consideration for the committee in such cases is whether patients need to be contacted to obtain consent, or whether it is acceptable to use the information for the new purpose without returning to the patient for further consent. The committee's decisions must be in accordance with applicable national law and conform to the requirements of this statement."*

VISCERAL involved the analysis of very large datasets of previously acquired and anonymized data, i.e. of already acquired datasets so that the above-mentioned problems for retrospective studies apply to the VISCERAL project. No additional procedures were conducted linked to the VISCERAL study, and all data were fully anonymized. The decision regarding the requirement of free informed consent procedures was dealt with by each local MEC, according to the relevant legislation.

3.2.3 Anonymization

All data used in the benchmarks are anonymized. Radiology reports were anonymized by removing all patient names, physician names, hospital and institution names and other identifying information. Radiology images were anonymized by blurring face regions in images/volumes that include this body area, removing any embedded text in the image, and locating and removing other identifying information such as serial numbers on implants.

3.2.4 Data Distribution During and After the Benchmarks

All medical data are sensitive by nature. In the context of VISCERAL, it is assured that all data are only available for non-commercial research use and only after signature of a user agreement that assures the use of the data in its given environment and for its research purpose. In VISCERAL, only registered participants can access the data and local copies of the data need to be destroyed after their use for research. The clauses of three ethics committees in Vienna, Barcelona and Heidelberg were taken into account to assure that data treatment is in line with all ethical guidelines. In VISCERAL, only anonymized data are shared in any case and thus all necessary steps are taken into account to assure privacy. The benchmarking campaigns are run in the cloud, in our case the cloud of Microsoft, called Azure (See also Chap. 2). Participants obtain a virtual machine and access to a data source after signing the user agreement with detailed user conditions and rules. All accesses to the virtual machines can be logged as can accesses to the data. Participants in the benchmark have access only to a small, manually controlled anonymous dataset. Very small subsets can also be made available for download in connection with the user agreement to get used to the data format and image types. The large test dataset, where the anonymization is less carefully controlled, is only accessible by the organizers. Clouds allow for storage of data in chosen geographical regions such as in Europe. This allows making sure that local storage and access rules can be verified and correspond to European legislation.

3.3 Relevant Legislation

All work on data collection of humans is conducted under the rules and legislation in place within the respective countries of the partners, which are based on the following:

- the Declaration of Helsinki (Informed consent for participation of human subjects in medical and scientific research, 2004) and the IHC (International conference on harmonization of technical requirements of pharmaceuticals for human use, Guideline for Good Clinical Practice (1996),
- European Directive 2001/20/EC (April 4, 2001) on Good Clinical Practice for clinical trials,
- Directive 95/46/EC of the European Parliament and of the Council of 24 October 1995 (amended 2003) on the protection of individuals with regard to the processing of personal data and on the free movement of such data,
- Regulation (CE) No 45/2001 of the European Parliament and of the Council of 18 December 2001, on the protection of individuals with regard to the processing of personal data by the institutions and bodies of the community and on the free movement of such data.

Furthermore, the Opinions of the European Group on Ethics in Science and New technologies (EGE) (specficially Opinion Nr.13 30/07/1999—Ethical issues of healthcare in the information society) are taken into account.

3.4 Procedures Implemented by Data Providers

Every partner who is data provider (GENCAT, MUW, and UKL-HD) is responsible for the compliance regarding the data contributed by this partner and informs for approval the local medical ethics committee (MEC)/institutional review board (IRB). These committees operate in accordance with international ethical guidelines and the national laws on medical research and protection of the human rights of subjects and privacy.

3.4.1 Agencia D'Informació, Avaluació i Qualitat en Salut, Spain

3.4.1.1 Requirements

Imaging data provided by the Agency to the VISCERAL project are a subset of an electronic health record, "Registre d'informaci sanitria de pacients" (Record of patient health information). Patient care is one of the reasons that allow recollection of personal health data, according to data protection laws. Additionally, the health record was declared by the Catalonian Health Department to the data protection authority (Declaration to the Data Protection Agency of Catalunya of the file "Registre d'informació sanitària de pacients", Record of patient health information). Research activities are included among the planned health record usage, and data may be submitted to research groups in the manner provided by the applicable laws. The main laws to be considered in order to transfer personal health information for research projects are as follows:

- ORGANIC LAW 15/1999 of 13 December on the Protection of Personal Data,
- Llei 21/2000, de 29 de desembre, sobre els drets d'informació concernent la salut i l'autonomia del pacient, i la documentació clínica (Patient's rights and clinical records), and
- LEY 14/2007, de 3 de julio, de Investigación biomédica (Biomedical Research).

According to these laws, in the absence of informed consent from patients, data may be submitted provided that it is effectively anonymized. If obtaining informed consent is not feasible, imaging data can be delivered after an anonymization process.

3.4.1.2 Final Status

The data transfer request was processed by the Department of Health in order to review the legal and ethical questions. No difficulties arose as a result of this reviewing process. Considering the amount of information in image files that could identify an individual or make him/her identifiable, a detailed analysis of the requirements for an effective anonymization of this information was carried out.

3.4.2 Medizinische Universität Wien (Austria)

3.4.2.1 Requirements

The Medical University of Vienna (MUW) provides anonymized medical imaging data to the project. As a general regulation, any study that involves human data such as VISCERAL conducted at MUW has to be approved by the medical ethics committee (Ethikkommission der Medizinischen Universität Wien,[1] EKMUW).

3.4.2.2   Final Status

At this point, EKMUW has approved the retrospective collection and the publication of anonymized medical imaging data in the course of the VISCERAL project and the involved evaluation. The basis for this decision was a study protocol providing detailed information regarding the study, the anonymization, the assurance of privacy and the data handling. The study protocol was an amendment to an existing protocol that covered the use of anonymized medical imaging data in the KHRESMOI project (Study protocol EK Nr.804/2010-Amendment December 2012). The amendment adds the collection of radiology report data and the publication of anonymized data for evaluation campaign purposes.

3.4.3   Universitätsklinikum Heidelberg (Germany)

3.4.3.1   Requirements

The Medical University of Heidelberg (UKL-HD) provides anonymized medical imaging data and corresponding reports to the project. As a general regulation, a study conducted at the UKL-HD has to be approved by the local ethics board (Ethikkommission der medizinischen Fakultät der Universität Heidelberg,[2] EKUKL-HD). The study must be conducted in accordance with Baden-Württemberg's Medical Association's professional code of conduct (Berufsordnung für Ärztinnen und Ärzte der Landesärztekammer Baden-Württemberg) in its current version. Patient names and all other confidential information are subject to the medical professional secrecy and the provisions of the Federal Data Privacy Act (Bundesdatenschutzgesetzes (BDSG)). A transfer of patient data happens only in anonymized form. Third persons get no insight into the original patient documents.

3.4.3.2   Final Status

The EKUKL-HD was consulted, and a study plan and an ethics proposal were reviewed. The retrospective collection and publication of anonymized medical imaging data in the course of the VISCERAL project and the involved evaluation are accepted under the following conditions:

---

[1]http://ethikkommission.meduniwien.ac.at/.
[2]http://www.medizinische-fakultaet-hd.uni-heidelberg.de/Ethikkommission.106025.0.html.

- Only datasets of patient of the age 18 or older are used.
- Retrospective datasets used are of the years 2005–2008, and an informed consent of these patients is not needed, because a retrospective obtention of informed consent would be extremely complex and elaborated without being certainly successful: probably, many patients are already deceased or cannot be contacted.
- In order to maintain further prospective datasets, medical imaging data collected during the clinical routine can be used only of patients (>18 years) that signed an informed consent to agree with the use of their images for the VISCERAL project.

The basis for the decision of the EKUKL-HD is the positive approval of the EKMUW, including a study protocol providing detailed information regarding the study, the anonymization, the assurance of privacy and the data handling, as well as a study protocol that covered the use of anonymized medical imaging data in the KHRESMOI project (Study protocol EK Nr.804/2010-Amendment December 2012).

3.5 Aspects, Recommendations and Conditions for Obtaining Approval from Ethical Committees

Out of the experience with the process of applying for an approval of the ethical boards of the UKL-HD and MUW, we gathered several aspects and recommendations that may help in similar future projects to deal with privacy questions and obtaining approval from ethical committees:

- **Age of patients included**: It may be helpful to only include datasets of patients of the age 18 or older.
- **Usage of retrospective versus prospective datasets**: In Germany, an informed consent by patients is needed. This means to contact every patient by telephone and/or by letter. In Heidelberg, there was the problem that we planned to use retrospective older datasets and that a retrospective obtention of informed consent was extremely complex and elaborated without being certainly successful, since it was probable that many patients were already deceased or moved because of the fact that the image data were out of a sample of patients being severely ill (cancer). Because of this, we obtained the approval to use retrospective older datasets (2005–2009) without informed consent of patients. Usage of prospective or current datasets is only permitted if an informed consent is signed, agreeing with the usage of the patient images and anonymized data for the project.
- **Anonymization of all data**: All selected image datasets were anonymized individually and locally by the three data providers. For anonymization, the following items were removed from the DICOM headers: date of birth (only age was preserved), institution name, patient name, patient ID, examination number and study date. A key of the patient ID and the referring pseudonym is held by the data provider and stored individually. Other metadata, such as clinical questions

and radiology reports, were anonymized, using only extracted RadLex terms (and their negations) from the reports. Additionally, whole-body CT scans were defaced (image data of the face were partly blurred), in order to ensure that no identification of a patient is possible.

- **End-User Agreement**: In order to ensure the correct and only scientific usage of the data, benchmark participants have to sign an end-user agreement. The signed agreements were checked and approved individually by Benchmark organizers.
- **Safe storage in the cloud**: VISCERAL Benchmarks are run on cloud servers, provided by Microsoft (Azure). Only authorized participants who signed the end-user agreements have access to the stored data. The data access closes when a benchmark is finished. Participants only have access to a small, well-chosen and anonymized dataset for training their algorithms. Since the cloud servers had to be in Europe, they are subject to European law. Access regulation and local data storage are secure and protected by European law.
- **Long-term usage of data**: A central element of sustainable, deep-impacting evaluation campaigns in developing new methods is the long-term availability of the data. VISCERAL aims at providing the data over a long period of time. Comparable datasets are the BRATS dataset for computer-based segmentation of brain lesions.[3] A deletion of the data after the end of the project would mean that the results of VISCERAL are not reproducible and can no longer be verified. In order to maintain the results and the scientific progress achieved through the project, the EKUKL-HD agreed to provide the data three more years after the end of the project. If further usage of the data is needed, an additional amendment for the corresponding study protocol will be provided.

3.6 Conclusion

Acquiring medical imaging research data in multicentre studies is not an easy process. All data acquisition requires that data privacy be respected and needs to be agreed upon by medical ethics commissions of the participating institutions. This chapter describes the steps that were taken in the VISCERAL project and some lessons learned to avoid delays in data acquisition that can also be useful for similar future projects. Safe storage and access of data in the cloud has a promising future for medical data analysis, as the risks of data misuse can be reduced in a straightforward way.

Acknowledgements The research leading to these results has received funding from the European Union Seventh Framework Programme (FP7/2007–2013) under grant agreement 318068 (VISCERAL).

---

[3]http://www2.imm.dtu.dk/projects/BRATS2012,https://vsd.unibe.ch/WebSite/BRATS2012/Start.

References

1. Hanbury A, Müller H, Langs G, Weber MA, Menze BH, Fernandez TS (2012) Bringing the algorithms to the data: cloud-based benchmarking for medical image analysis. In: Catarci T, Forner P, Hiemstra D, Peñas A, Santucci G (eds) CLEF 2012. LNCS, vol 7488. Springer, Heidelberg, pp 24–29. doi:10.1007/978-3-642-33247-0_3
2. Langs G, Hanbury A, Menze B, Müller H (2013) VISCERAL: towards large data in medical imaging — challenges and directions. In: Greenspan H, Müller H, Syeda-Mahmood T (eds) MCBR-CDS 2012. LNCS, vol 7723. Springer, Heidelberg, pp 92–98. doi:10.1007/978-3-642-36678-9_9
3. Jiménez-del Toro OA, Müller H, Krenn M, Gruenberg K, Taha AA, Winterstein M, Eggel I, Foncubierta-Rodríguez A, Goksel O, Jakab A, Kontokotsios G, Langs G, Menze B, Salas Fernandez T, Schaer R, Walleyo A, Weber MA, Dicente Cid Y, Gass T, Heinrich M, Jia F, Kahl F, Kechichian R, Mai D, Spanier AB, Vincent G, Wang C, Wyeth D, Hanbury A (2016) Cloud-based evaluation of anatomical structure segmentation and landmark detection algorithms: visceral anatomy benchmarks. IEEE Trans Med Imaging 35(11):2459
4. Krenn M, Dorfer M, Jiménez del Toro OA, Müller H, Menze B, Weber MA, Hanbury A, Langs G (2016) Creating a large-scale silver corpus from multiple algorithmic segmentations. In: Menze B, Langs G, Montillo A, Kelm M, Müller H, Zhang S, Cai W, Metaxas D (eds) MCV 2015. LNCS, vol 9601. Springer, Cham, pp 103–115. doi:10.1007/978-3-319-42016-5_10
5. World Medical Association Declaration of Helsinki (2001) Ethical principles for medical research involving human subjects. Bull World Health Organ 79(4):373
6. Elger B, Iavindrasana J, Lo Iacono L, Müller H, Roduit N, Summers P, Wright J (2010) Strategies for health data exchange for secondary, cross-institutional clinical research. Comput Methods Programs Biomed 99(3):230–251
7. Hughes J, Hunter D, Sheehan M, Wilkinson S, Wrigley A (2010) European textbook on ethics in research. Publications Office of the European Union, Luxembourg
8. Tassé AM, Budin-Ljøsne I, Knoppers BM, Harris JR (2010) Retrospective access to data: the ENGAGE consent experience. Eur J Hum Genet 18(7):741–745
9. Vayena E, Ganguli-Mitra A, Biller-Andorno N (2013) Guidelines on biobanks: emerging. Ethical issues in governing biobanks: global perspectives. Ashgate Publishing, Farnham, pp 23–35
10. Declaration on ethical considerations regarding health databases (2002) WMA General Assembly, Washington (s 1)

Chapter 4
Annotating Medical Image Data

**Katharina Grünberg, Oscar Jimenez-del-Toro, Andras Jakab,
Georg Langs, Tomàs Salas Fernandez, Marianne Winterstein,
Marc-André Weber and Markus Krenn**

Abstract This chapter describes the annotation of the medical image data that were used in the VISCERAL project. Annotation of regions in the 3D images is non-trivial, and tools need to be chosen to limit the manual work and have semi-automated annotation available. For this, several tools that were available free of charge or with limited costs were tested and compared. The GeoS tool was finally chosen for the annotation based on the detailed analysis, allowing for efficient and effective annotations. 3D slice was chosen for smaller structures with low contrast to complement the annotations. A detailed quality control was also installed, including an automatic tool that attributes organs to annotate and volumes to specific annotators, and then compares results. This allowed to judge the confidence in specific annotators and also to iteratively refine the annotation instructions to limit the subjectivity of the task as much as possible. For several structures, some subjectivity remains and this was measured via double annotations of the structure. This allows the judgement of the quality of automatic segmentations.

Source code is available at:
https://github.com/Visceral-Project/annotationTicketingFramework

K. Grünberg · M. Winterstein · M.-A. Weber
University of Heidelberg, Heidelberg, Germany
e-mail: katharina.gruenberg@med.uni-heidelberg.de

O. Jimenez-del-Toro (✉)
University of Applied Sciences Western Switzerland (HES–SO), Sierre, Switzerland
e-mail: oscar.jimenez@hevs.ch

A. Jakab · G. Langs · M. Krenn
Medical University of Vienna, Vienna, Austria
e-mail: georg.langs@meduniwien.ac.at

T. Salas Fernandez
Agencia D'Informció, Avaluació i Qualitat en Salut, Catalonia, (GENCAT), Spain

© The Author(s) 2017
A. Hanbury et al. (eds.), *Cloud-Based Benchmarking
of Medical Image Analysis*, DOI 10.1007/978-3-319-49644-3_4

4.1 Introduction

Since during clinical routine, only a very small portion of the increasing amounts of medical imaging data are used for helping diagnosis, the VISCERAL (Visual Concept Extraction Challenge in Radiology) project aimed at providing the necessary data for developing clinical image assessment algorithms. An objective was to conduct Benchmarks for identifying successful computational strategies. The VISCERAL project developed a cloud-based infrastructure for the evaluation of detection, analysis and retrieval algorithms on large medical image datasets [8, 9]. VISCERAL organized benchmarks to exploit and compare multiple state-of-the-art solutions designed for image segmentation, landmark localization and retrieval [13]. The VISCERAL Anatomy Benchmarks focused on automatic identification, localization and segmentation of organs in image volumes. An anatomical reference annotation dataset, the Gold Corpus, was created for these Benchmarks using CT (computed tomography) and MRI (magnetic resonance imaging) volumes annotated with up to 20 organs and 53 landmarks each.

One goal of the VISCERAL project was to create a large dataset containing high-quality expert annotations in medical imaging data (i.e. organ segmentations, landmark localizations and lesion annotations). For this purpose, various manual and semi-automatic segmentation tools were evaluated in the search for fast and effective 3D annotation software interfaces that can reduce the time spent and workload of the radiologist making the manual segmentations and annotations of the structures. A ticketing framework was also developed to facilitate the management of multiple annotation types, the distribution of annotation tickets to multiple annotators and the implementation of a quality control procedure to ensure consistent annotation quality across annotators. This chapter describes the two selected annotation tools, the framework that was built to monitor and distribute annotation tickets, the typical life cycle of an annotation ticket, detailed annotation guidelines for the annotators and the procedure of determining the inter-annotator agreement.

4.2 3D Annotation Software

With the ever-increasing amount of patient data generated in hospitals and the need to support a patient diagnosis with these data, computerized automatic and semi-automatic algorithms are a promising option in the clinical field [6]. An initial step in the development of such systems for diagnosis aid is to have manually annotated datasets that are used to train and implement machine-learning methods to mimic a human annotator. The manual segmentation of the patients' 3D volumes is commonly used for radiology imaging in order to separate various structures in the images and allow processing tissue of the structures separately. Manual segmentation, on the other hand, demands an intensive and time-consuming labour from the radiologists.

Variation and errors in the segmentations are common, depending on the experience of the annotator [12].

Several tools have been developed for the manual and semi-automatic segmentation of anatomical structures and annotation of pathologies present in medical imaging [3, 4, 10, 12, 14]. The implemented segmentation methods range from simple manual outlining in 2D cross sections to more elaborated solutions, like deformable registration that finds spatial correspondences between 3D images and a labelled atlas [12]. An important feature of manual or semi-automatic segmentation methods is that they assist the radiologists in the final decision of the resulting 3D structures [7]. Some of these tools are added to application frameworks that provide visualization and image analysis for an integral medical image computing experience.

An objective of the VISCERAL project was to take advantage of effective user-friendly annotation tools that can reduce the time necessary for annotations and segmentations in a multimodal imaging dataset (MRI, CT). Visualization frameworks are also available that reduce the time to develop new applications through the combinations of algorithms, which is usually faster than writing code [1, 2]. Various available tools were explored for the selection of the tool used for the annotation tasks in the VISCERAL project. The selected annotation tool had to make annotations in CT and MRI images acquired with a variety of scanners and in different MR sequences such as T1 weighted and T2 FLAIR, and with a resolution of the annotated voxels of 1 cm or lower. To ensure sustainability, tools with at least a minimum of support were preferred. These requirements further include adaptability of the included segmentation method to overcome the differences in image contrast and resolution in the dataset.

A brief description of the medical annotation functionality of the evaluated tools is presented in the following sections. The criteria used for selecting the definitive tool are also mentioned. Finally, the description of the methods and use of the proposed tools are discussed. The selected tools allowed the radiologists to segment 20 relevant structures of 15 organs in the human body, identify up to 53 landmarks and detect pathological lesions in full-body patient scans. Both individual voxels and homogeneous regions were labelled in the 3D volumes of the dataset. Medical raw data to be annotated were in the DICOM (Digital Imaging and Communications in Medicine) format. The raw DICOM files were converted into NIfTI (Neuroimaging Informatics Technology Initiative) format, because this is a widely used and accepted format that significantly reduces the file size in case of large 3D data. Both the image data and the resulting volume annotations were used in the NIfTI format.

4.2.1 Evaluation Criteria

A list of ten criteria was defined for the comparison between the tools. The goal was to evaluate their main functionality applied to the annotation tasks needed for the creation of the VISCERAL Gold Corpus. The criteria chosen to compare the available annotation tools were as follows:

- ability to perform 3D annotation in CT and MRI volumes;
- flexibility to segment different structures and points of interest;
- user-friendly segmentation method;
- optimal visualization of the medical images and segmentations;
- effectiveness of the segmentation;
- interactive user corrections in the semi-automatic output;
- time spent in a complete structure segmentation;
- adaptability to data obtained from different scanners and image contrasts;
- format of the output segmentations;
- upgrading of the tool with minimum technical support during and after the project has ended.

4.2.2   Reviewed Annotation Tools

For the selection of the VISCERAL annotation tool, the visualization and application frameworks that are already available free of charge were evaluated. The frameworks had to contain a semi-automatic segmentation tool that could reduce the time required for making manual annotations of 3D structures and points of interest. Six frameworks with no license fees: GeoS [4], ITK-SNAP [14], ImageJ, MeVisLab, MITK and 3D Slicer [11], were included in the study. Some Web-based applications with annotation functionality available such as [10] are limited to a specific application or image analysis type, making them unfit to be used for the VISCERAL project multistructure annotation task. Other available frameworks such as SciRun,[1] Osirix[2] and Volview[3] were also reviewed but were discarded early in the selection process.

4.2.2.1   3D Slicer

3D Slicer[4] is a module-based software where each module performs a particular image processing task. There are two modules that can be useful for segmenting and annotating medical 3D images. The first is called Simple Region Growing Segmentation and it is based on intensity statistics. After choosing a desired number of fiducials in the region of interest, it applies ITK filters for curvature flow and connected confidence producing a 2-class segmentation. The segmentations can be improved by increasing the number of iterations, the multiplier and the neighbourhood radius options. More than one fiducial or seed is allowed for refinement of the output. The other module included is EMSegment Easy that performs a quick intensity-based image segmentation on MRI. The user defines the volumes to be

---

[1]http://www.sci.utah.edu/cibc-software/scirun.html.

[2]http://www.osirix-viewer.com.

[3]http://www.kitware.com/opensource/volview.html.

[4]http://www.slicer.org.

segmented, specifies the number of structures and can add additional subclasses of the structures. Samples are taken from the structures of interest to define the intensity distribution and the weighting of a node in the tree. Once the algorithm is run, the target images are segmented and the label map with corresponding statistics is returned [11].

4.2.2.2 GeoS

The Microsoft medical image analysis project InnerEye focuses on the automatic analysis of the patients' scans. Its annotation tool GeoS[5] has an algorithm to efficiently segment 3D images using a geodesic symmetric filter with contrast-sensitive spatial smoothness. Its behaviour is comparable to that of graph cut algorithms but with a much faster implementation. The segmentation method is based on a generalized geodesic distance transform (GGDT). A geodesic distance map is initialized from a soft seed mask. The seed region is determined interactively. It uses different brush strokes to quickly indicate a foreground object and the background that surrounds it. In this matter, geodesic distance is described as the distance between two points in an image that takes into account image contents such as intensity gradients. One of the most sought-after requirements is edge-sensitivity whereby the image processing system is able to change its behaviour depending on the local image contrast. This tool is able to perform contrast-sensitive image editing or processing. It shares some of the image processing tasks unifying previously diverse image techniques in such a manner that at least some processing may be shared so that computational resource requirements can be reduced.

4.2.2.3 ITK-SNAP

ITK-SNAP[6] is a software application that provides a set of tools for segmenting medical images' volumetric data. The software provides both an algorithm referred to as "Snake evolution" and a visualization interface for 3D image segmentation. The contour evolution on which its algorithm is based uses the image gradient information and the global intensity to expand or constrain the contour with respect to user given seed points. It provides a segmentation pipeline in three steps with three modifiable parameters that influence the output of the segmentation: balloon force, curvature force and advection force. These three parameters regulate the region growing expansion of the segmentation and the smoothness of the output borders. The framework includes a wizard for image upload and also a polygon tool that allows the user to perform freehand annotation. The freehand annotation tool can be expressed in either a continuous curve or piecewise linear with an adjustable segment length.

---

[5]http://research.microsoft.com/en-us/projects/geos.
[6]http://www.itksnap.org.

4.2.2.4 ImageJ

ImageJ[7] contains several image segmentation algorithms based on intensity range thresholds. In particular, the Robust Automatic Threshold Selection (RATS) performs a threshold on previously established regions using a recursive quad-tree architecture. It calculates the sum of the original voxels weighted by the gradient pixels. Other plug-ins such as the watershed algorithm are available for segmenting images but they mostly rely on histogram thresholding and Gaussian modelling of the intensity values in the images, which can provide an initial estimate but has to be completed by the user with freehand 2D slice-by-slice manual annotation.

4.2.2.5 MeVisLab

MeVisLab[8] is an integrated development environment with a modular framework that allows developing image processing algorithms and visualization and interaction methods. It is possible to create an end-user application with a network composed of modules based on Open Inventor scene graphs, OpenGL, ITK, VTK and SDK. It supports DICOM files as well as NIfTI formats. Conversion of one format to the other is also included within the available modules. Although there are few segmentation algorithms outside those available in the ITK and VTK libraries, the user can use LiveWire combined with freehand manual annotation on a slice-by-slice basis. LiveWire is a graph cut algorithm where the user can adjust the gradient, Laplacian and directional weighting. There is also a "bulge" module that can easily bend, expand and contract manual annotations with the mouse.

4.2.2.6 MITK

The Medical Imaging Interaction Toolkit (MITK)[9] was created as a software system for development of interactive medical image processing software. It implements both ITK and VTK libraries but also offers additional development and interactive features of its own like 3D-synchronized multiviewer layout. It contains various segmentation methods based on threshold functions such as the Otsu segmentation where it is possible to define a number of regions based on a Gaussian modelling of the intensity value image histograms. It is also possible to apply a region growing algorithm with a user-given seed. The framework only allows one seed per region and freehand wiping, correction and filling of the created segmentation. Another option when manual 2D slice segmentations are available is to interpolate the missing slices and create a surface of a structure of interest.

---

[7]http://rsb.info.nih.gov/ij.

[8]http://www.mevislab.de.

[9]http://www.mitk.org.

Table 4.1 Report on the evaluation criteria for each of the frameworks or annotation tools

GeoS	ImageJ	ITK-SNAP	MeVisLab	MITK	3DSlicer	Evaluation Criteria
+	+	+	+	+	+	Annotation on 3D volumes (CT and MRI)
+	-	+	+	+	+	Semi-automatic segmentation method different shapes flexibility
+	-	o	+	o	+	Segmentation user-friendly usage
o	o	+	+	+	+	Optimal image visualization of segmentation
+	-	o	+	+	+	Effectiveness in VISCERAL data of the segmentation method
+	+	+	+	+	+	Interactive output corrections
+	o	+	-	o	o	Semi-automatic algorithm time reduction vs. manual annotation
+	-	o	-	+	+	Local image contrast flexibility
+	o	o	-	+	o	Output annotation format
+	-	-	-	o	o	Upgrading of the tool

+: Satisfactory   o: Insufficient   -: Missing

4.2.3   Tool Comparison

In this section, we discuss how each of the considered tools satisfies the evaluation criteria. Table 4.1 summarizes the evaluation of the frameworks and annotation tools for each of the evaluation criteria listed in Sect. 4.2.1.

4.2.3.1   Compatible 3D Annotation on CT and MRI Volumes

ITK-SNAP and ImageJ ask for a greyscale or RGB image when they upload and ITK-SNAP uses a wizard for loading a file. Intensity values with an intensity precision larger than 16-bit are approximated. MeVisLab can upload DICOM volumes and Analyze-formatted files but NIfTI files are not supported. Both MITK and 3D Slicer can upload a wide range of different image formats and contain converting format functions. GeoS does not support DICOM files but works with NIfTI files as well as other image formats such as Analyze and Tagged Image File Format.

4.2.3.2   Flexibility to Segment Different Structures and Points of Interest

Tools that allow freehand annotation such as MeVisLab, ImageJ and MITK can be adapted to structures with different shapes and make modifications on 2D views of the generated volumes. ITK-SNAP and region growing algorithms like the ones in 3D Slicer and GeoS depend on the number of seeds for their adaptation to the particular shape features of the organs. All of the selected frameworks are not limited to a particular application and can perform segmentations on different organs and points of interest.

4.2.3.3   User-Friendly Segmentation Method Usage

The semi-automatic segmentation method sought by VISCERAL needs to be easy to apply and must be performed in real time in order to allow for optimal user interaction. Segmentation methods like those used in ImageJ and ITK-SNAP require an initial trial and error user interaction to define the best values of the parameters involved. It can take the users some time to understand the functionality of these parameters when they are not familiar with them, as is likely the case for the annotators of the Gold Corpus. The GeoS tool has a fast, straightforward algorithm that can easily be used by the users, and the default parameters given by the tool can be used without need for modification for most of the structures. Adding seed points in the MeVisLab and 3D Slicer region growing algorithms is also a simple task once it is combined with freehand manual corrections.

4.2.3.4   Optimal Visualization of Segmentation and Medical Images

The ImageJ framework has an independent window visualization that requires the handling of multiple open windows and manual interaction for the user to navigate in 3D medical images. MITK and 3D Slicer have a better visualization of the data with the three views visible at the same time and a multiplanar 3D representation or volume rendering that the user can zoom in and out, rotate and navigate with the mouse. One drawback in MITK is that changing between images can cause losing the defined orientation of the image requiring the user to reset the desired image location for visualization. The GeoS tool has a simple, easy-to-use interface with the three views in which it is possible to make annotations. Unfortunately, volume rendering is still not supported and the segmentations can only be visualized in 2D in each view.

4.2.3.5   Effectiveness of the Segmentation

The purpose of selecting frameworks with semi-automatic segmentation methods is to reduce the amount of work when making the annotations and allowing the radiologists to add their experience and input in the segmentations. Since all of the selected tools are not application oriented to a single type of anatomical structure, they can obtain accurate segmentations with enough user feedback. ImageJ and MeVisLab have the least evolved segmentation methods while ITK-SNAP, 3D Slicer and GeoS are the best annotation tools to perform semi-automatic segmentations in medical images.

4.2.3.6 Easy Interaction with the User for Corrections in the Semi-automatic Output

Most of the application frameworks contain the option to cut or add new voxels to the segmentation output in 2D slices if the segmentation has leakage or a part is missing. Other tools such as GeoS can improve the segmentations by adding more strokes either in the background or in the foreground from the structure of interest. Once the algorithm is run again, it provides a new segmentation incorporating user input influencing the full 3D volume of the segmentation. This is useful for rapid visual inspection of the results and minor user interaction in any of the views for corrections in the output. Updating small changes however still requires the algorithm to be run fully, even though it has a fast implementation for the whole structure and no freehand correction tool is available in the current GeoS version.

4.2.3.7 Time Required for Complete Structure Segmentation

The GeoS annotation tool is the fastest tool for segmenting a complete structure because of its "lazy annotation" implementation, the good data visualization and the annotation in the three views at the same time. ITK-SNAP and multiple seed algorithms like those in MeVisLab and 3D Slicer can also provide quick segmentations that may need user interaction to correct some leakage or missing parts in the segmented volume. For the other available options, there are efficient algorithms to start the segmentation process but eventually they require manual freehand improvements to refine the segmentations and this can take some time, especially for structures with low intensity contrast and soft edges.

4.2.3.8 Segmentation Method Flexibility to Data Obtained from Different Scanners and Image Contrasts

Some of the segmentation methods that involve thresholding can be very sensitive to image noise and full image contrast of the different structures. A more local definition of the contrast is desired, particularly in MRI where field inhomogeneities are common and intensity values can change significantly even within the same structure. An advantage of the GeoS tool and the ITK-SNAP methods is their local approach that limits the expansion of the segmentations to a specific region. One limitation in the ITK-SNAP method is that it is limited to changes in the image gradient and it can also be affected by image noise and poor soft tissue contrast.

4.2.3.9   Output Format of the Annotations

MeVisLab generates contour segmentation object lists from the segmentation results that have to be converted to a different format for their inclusion in the annotation analysis backend. With 3D Slicer, the user can decide the label of each structure and add subclasses of it. Only in the GeoS tool and the MITK framework, the output of the segmentations can be saved in a NIfTI format without additional plug-ins in accordance with the data format definition for the Gold Corpus annotation for VISCERAL. In addition, the RadLex terminology is expected to already be included in the final version of the GeoS prototype, which makes the annotations comparable and provides a better set-up for long-term use of the annotations.

4.2.3.10   Upgrading of the Tool with Minimum User Support
for Its Availability During and After the Project Has Ended

Due to the close collaboration with Microsoft and their interest in supporting medical imaging projects, the GeoS tool was adapted and improved based on various requests. Other frameworks such as MITK, 3D Slicer, and ImageJ can be upgraded using freely available plug-ins. However, their maintenance and specific adaptation for the VISCERAL requirements would have involved significantly more effort from the project consortium.

4.2.4   Selected Software and Technical Aspects

The final decision was made in collaboration with physicians evaluating the considered tools and comparing their usefulness. The Microsoft GeoS annotation tool was selected as the principal annotation tool mainly because of its efficiency and accuracy in the segmentations, which require only a few brush strokes from the user to run segmentations in 3D volumes respecting strong edges. Other advantages over the remaining tools are the tool simplicity and easy-to-use annotation interface with the learning of only a few key presses needed to start using the tool for annotations. 3D Slicer was selected as the secondary annotation tool.

For the organ annotations, in general the GeoS software was used, providing means to an interactive, semi-automated segmentation. Nevertheless, for whole-body MRI (T1w and T2w), where structures such as the vertebrae, the kidneys, the pancreas or certain muscles are only visible from a few coronal slices, the 3D Slicer software was used, since GeoS does not support the annotation of point-like structures. In the following sections, we briefly describe the annotation process in GeoS and 3D Slicer.

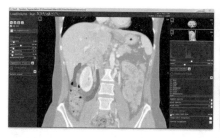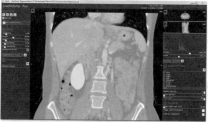

Fig. 4.1 Segmentation method: with only a foreground stroke for the kidney (*yellow*) and two background strokes for the surrounding organs (*red, left image*), an initial segmentation of the kidney is obtained (*right image*). This segmentation can be further refined with more strokes

4.2.4.1 GeoS

By clicking "LoadVolume" on the initial screen, the user selects the assigned image file to be annotated. The segmentation can be started with only a few strokes in the desired structure (foreground) pressing Shift and a left mouse drag (Fig. 4.1, marked yellow). To limit the extension of the segmentation, strokes outside the structure (background) were created with Shift and right mouse drag (Fig. 4.1, marked red). For better automated segmentation, foreground strokes were put in all three views. The segmentation process is then started. The created segment could then be improved by adding more strokes in the structure and in the background and by running the segmentation process again. Five-to-ten iterations were needed to have a good match of the created segmentation with the anatomical structure in the volume. The segmentation tool has five modifiable parameters: iterations, margin, gamma, pre-smoothing and post-smoothing. For most of the segmentations, a margin of 10 and a gamma of 1 were used. For large organs, such as the liver or the lung, the margin was reduced. For the other parameters, the default presets were used. Finally, the created annotations were saved in separate NIfTI files without modifying the original images. In this way, the annotation for one whole-body volume was completed in 3–4 h. A few examples of segmented annotations from various organs are shown in Fig. 4.2.

4.2.4.2 3D Slicer

The DICOM volumes are loaded into the software and the Annotation Module is used to annotate structures of interest. The landmarks within the patient coordinate system are then saved and exported in text files.

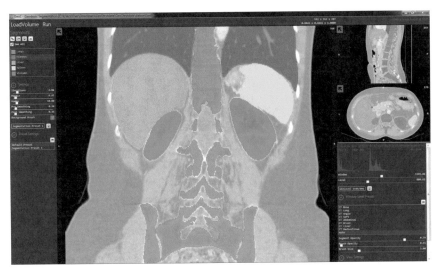

Fig. 4.2 Annotation example of different structures in an abdominal CT

4.3 VISCERAL Ticketing Tool/Framework

Manually annotating organs or landmarks in images is a complex process involving
many participants, including the administrators of the process, the experts that do
the annotation and the experts responsible for quality control. In the VISCERAL
project, a system was developed to simplify the management of the manual annotation
process. It is based on the commonly used process from software engineering of
assigning *tickets* to people for tasks that should be done, where the status of the
completion of each assigned task can be tracked. For medical image annotation, an
annotation ticket is assigned to an annotator requesting the segmentation of a specific
organ or identification of landmarks in a specific image. The VISCERAL ticketing
framework is designed to monitor and manage the full life cycle of an annotation
ticket, to provide an interface for annotators and quality control (QC) team members
for ticket submission. The framework consists of three main components:

1. Ticketing Database: A MySQL database that stores information of volumes to
   annotate, annotators, annotation types, tickets and their states (pending, submitted, QC passed and QC failed).
2. Backend: A backend implemented in MATLAB, to manage volumes, annotators,
   ticket types and annotation tickets. The backend is used to distribute tickets,
   to perform automated quality checks and to distribute QC tickets of submitted
   annotations.
3. Frontend: A Web interface that is used by annotators and QC team members to
   receive their assigned tickets and to submit annotations and QC results.

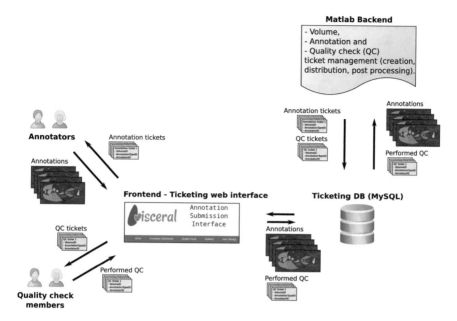

Fig. 4.3 Workflow overview of the VISCERAL ticketing framework

Figure 4.3 provides an overview of the ticketing system implemented within the VISCERAL project. The framework source code is available,[10] which provides create statements for the ticketing DB, the source of the Web interface, getter and setter functions of the backend implemented in Matlab including a tutorial and installation guidelines to set up the framework. The interface is designed using Java.

4.3.1 Ticketing System Database

The database (DB) of the ticketing system is created by SQL scripts provided in the ticketing repository. All relevant information is stored in five DB tables:

- **Annotator**: Identified by an AnnotatorID, holds next to contact information, name and password (for login) a flag indicating if the annotator is currently available and an additional flag if the annotator is considered a QC team member.
- **Volume**: A volume is identified by its PatientID and VolumeID. Additionally, the modality, body region and the filename are stored.
- **AnnotationType**: Entries in this table define which types of annotations can be managed by the ticketing system. Each entry is identified by its AnnotationTypeID. Additionally, the name, the file extension of the submitted files, the remote upload

---

[10]https://github.com/Visceral-Project/annotationTicketingFramework.

directory, the category (segmentation, landmarks,...) and an optional string describing the files prefix are stored. Exemplary entries of this table are created within the given SQL scripts.

- **Status**: Defines all states a ticket can have during its life cycle. A status is identified by its StatusID and stores its name and description as well as to which type of annotators (QC and normal annotators) the status option is available in the ticketing Web interface. Default entries of this table are created within the given SQL scripts.
- **Annotation**: This table represents an annotation ticket. An annotation entry is identified by its PatientID and VolumeID, the AnnotationTypeID, the StatusID and the AnnotatorID of the annotator to whom a ticket is assigned. Additionally, the filename, a timestamp, the ID of the annotator who performs the QC of the ticket and a QC comment are stored for each ticket.

Figure 4.4 illustrates the ER (entity relationship) diagram of the resulting database.

4.3.2   Annotation Ticket Life Cycle

The typical life cycle of an annotation ticket within the VISCERAL project can be outlined as follows:

1. Creation of an annotation list with the annotations that need to be done (tickets) and its upload to the Web interface.
2. The Web interface has a login user name and password for each of the annotators.
3. The annotator ID is used in the naming of the tickets:
   subjectXX acquisitionZZ[modalityYY] RadLexID annotatorID:nii
4. The annotators upload their files next to the ticket and the name of the file is implemented to be the same as the ticket for their backend analysis.
5. All the annotations are saved in the same folder to download them and use them in the analysis.
6. The annotation backend produces a new list of tickets for the new annotations needed and from which annotators.
7. The list in the interface is updated.
8. Depending on the type of annotation, an automated quality check is performed to detect common annotation errors, such as empty label volumes, incorrect file extensions or wrong naming of landmarks.
9. If the annotation passes the automated quality check, the ticket is assigned to a quality control (QC) annotator; otherwise, it is reassigned to the annotator for corrections to the annotation.
10. The QC annotator receives the QC ticket through the Web interface, performs the QC and submits the QC result (including textual feedback if the QC is negative) through the Web interface.

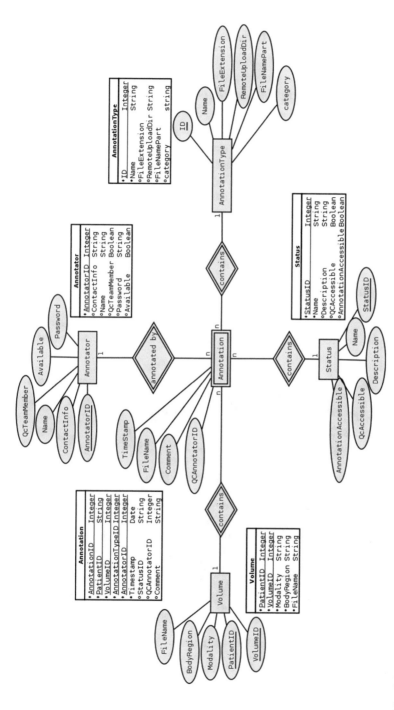

Fig. 4.4 Entity relationship diagram of the VISCERAL Ticketing System DB

11. The ticket reaches its final state if the QC is positive; otherwise, the annotator receives textual feedback and the ticket is reassigned for annotation.
12. The annotators receive their new set of tickets when they login.

4.3.3 Manual Annotation Instructions

In order to ensure reproducible annotations from multiple annotators, detailed instructions on the annotation of each organ were created. These annotation instructions describe the specificities of performing the anatomical structure segmentations and landmark locations of the Gold Corpus, complete with illustrations. To reduce the probability of misunderstandings, the instructions were written in the native language of the radiologists doing the annotation (in this case Hungarian). Below, we describe some aspects that need to be made explicit in the annotation instructions and show some of the example images.

4.3.3.1 Organ Segmentation

When delineating the organs, we face the problem of defining the outer extensions of the structure, requiring a definition of what part of a connected structure is still

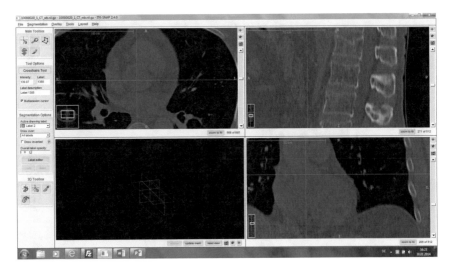

Fig. 4.5 Instructions for segmenting the aorta beginning in whole-body CTs: in the above *left* window, an axial slice is shown and the cross wires are centred at the aortic bulb in the height of the aortic valve. The below *right* window shows a coronary slice. The cross wire is located in the aortic bulb. You should segment until you see the diameter of aorta in the axial slices being in the region of aortic bulb and you could control that on the coronary slice

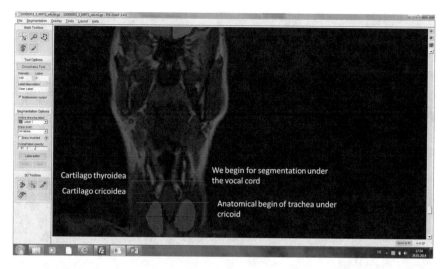

Fig. 4.6 Coronal whole-body MRI T1 weighted of the head/neck demonstrating the beginning of the trachea: the anatomical beginning of the trachea is under the cricoids, but that is not suitable for manual segmentation, so we define the beginning of trachea for segmentation under the vocal cord. Trachea (*purple*) and thyroid gland (*blue*)

"within" the organ and what is already "outside" of the organ, belonging to a different structure (that may or may not be in the list of annotated organs). Some organs, such as the lungs, liver and kidneys, have a hilum, which is a depression or indentation where vessels and nerves enter. It must be explicitly specified how to handle the hilum in the manual annotation — we specified that the hilum has to be cut off during the segmentation process. It is also often useful to provide an "algorithm" for the annotator to follow, as illustrated in Figs. 4.5 and 4.6. Some examples of organ segmentations are shown in Fig. 4.7.

4.3.3.2   Landmark Location

Anatomical landmarks are the locations of selected anatomical structures that can be identified in images of multiple modalities, such as CT or MRI, unenhanced or enhanced scans, whole-body images or with limited field of view. Their universal nature makes them important as a first step in parsing image content, or for triangulating other more specific anatomical structures. Overall, 40 landmarks were selected to be identified. Examples of annotated landmarks are shown in Fig. 4.8.

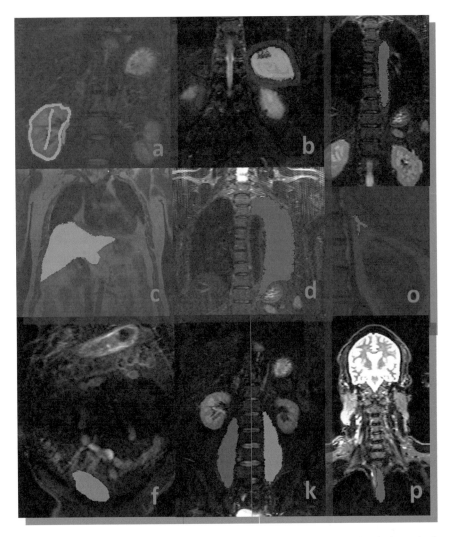

Fig. 4.7 Examples of organ segmentation in MRI T1w and T1w. **a** Kidney: Marked *grey* is the foreground stroke for the liver. Marked *red* is the background stroke defining the border of the organ. **b** Spleen. **c** Liver. **d** Lung (*left*). **f** M. rectus abdominis (*right*). **k** M. psoas major. **n** Aorta. **o** Adrenal gland. **p** Trachea

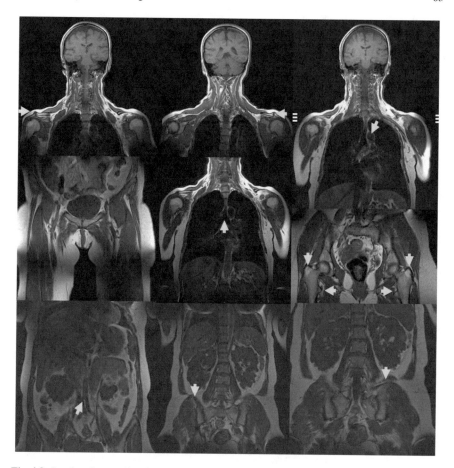

Fig. 4.8 Landmark examples. From *right top* to *left bottom*: *right* and *left* lateral end of the clavicle, tip of aortic arch, symphysis below, tracheal bifurcation, trochanter major at the tip and trochanter minor (most medal part), aortic bifurcation, Crista iliaca (at the *top*)

4.4   Inter-annotator Agreement

To analyse the reliability of Gold Corpus annotations, the agreement of different experts was investigated by comparing multiple annotations of a specific structure obtained from multiple annotators. The similarity of two annotations for this purpose is measured using the Dice coefficient [5], which is a spatial overlap measure that is 1 for perfect overlap and 0 if no overlap of two segmentations is present. The Dice coefficient, also called the overlap index, is the most frequently used metric in validating medical volume segmentations. Zou et al. [15] used the Dice coefficient as a measure of the reproducibility as a statistical validation of manual annotation where segmentors repeatedly annotated the same image [13]. In this context, inter-annotator agreements are reported independently for each structure in each modality

Table 4.2 Inter-annotator agreements of structures and modalities addressed within VISCERAL

Structure	CT Wb	CT-ce Thx/Abd	MRT1 Wb	MRT1 cefs-Abd
Lung R	0.974	0.946	0.925	
Lung L	0.971	0.945	0.902	
Kidney R	0.889	0.937	0.917	0.908
Kidney L	0.921	0.929	0.909	0.865
Liver	0.950	0.965	0.891	0.932
Spleen	0.946	0.934	0.685	0.925
Urinary Bladder	0.875	0.933	0.842	0.819
Psoas Major R	0.840	0.854	0.836	0.823
Psoas Major L	0.847	0.848	0.849	0.802
Trachea	0.894	0.877	0.768	
Aorta	0.884	0.856	0.849	0.768
Sternum	0.891	0.810		
1st Lumbar Vertebra	0.811	0.914	0.744	0.546
Muscle Body of Rectus Abdominis R	0.811	0.709		
Muscle Body of Rectus Abdominis L	0.734	0.637		
Pancreas	0.615	0.785	**0.486**	0.639
Gallbladder	0.689	0.857	0.742	
Thyroid Gland	0.658	0.781		
Adrenal Gland R	**0.347**	0.671	**0.465**	**0.305**
Adrenal Gland L	**0.485**	0.743	0.545	**0.338**

of the Gold Corpus and are obtained by comparing Gold Corpus segmentations from different annotators to additionally performed segmentations of the same structures in the same volumes (double annotations). Inter-annotator agreement is finally derived by averaging the Dice coefficients of all double annotations performed for a specific structure and modality and are shown in Table 4.2. Missing values are due to the structure being out of field such as the trachea in MRT1cefs-abdominal volumes (MRT T1 weighted contrast-enhanced sequence with fat saturation of the abdomen) or bad contrast of the addressed structure in a certain modality.

Organs such as the adrenal glands show, depending on the annotated modality, a Dice coefficient smaller than 0.5 (see the bold values in Table 4.2). The reason for this is probably that the adrenal glands have the best contrast in contrast-enhanced CT compared to other sequences. The CT volumes have overall the best average Dice coefficients also in small anatomical structures such as the adrenal glands. The adrenal glands, the thyroid gland, the pancreas and the bodies of the rectus abdominis muscles have the smallest average Dice coefficients which are smaller and/or equal than 0.8 in all four modalities: in whole-body CT and MRI (T1 weighted), in contrast-enhanced CT of thorax and abdomen and in contrast-enhanced and fat-saturated T1-weighted MRI. The contrast-enhanced CT sequence is the best for the adrenal glands, the thyroid gland and the pancreas. The reason for that is a worse contrast in the other sequences at the adrenal gland regions, especially at the right one in a small window between liver, right kidney and vertebral column in the fatty tissue. For the bodies of the rectus abdominis muscle, the native whole-body CT sequence is ahead, probably due to a better contrast for this structure without contrast media. If the muscle bodies of the rectus abdominis are small, the contrast between fatty tissue and muscle is also not sufficient to reliably and repeatably segment these structures. The difference of the pancreatic tissue and the fat-surrounding tissue is not high enough without contrast media and therefore difficult to annotate. Figure 4.9 visualizes the agreement between two annotators based on a liver segmentation in a contrast-enhanced CT volume of the thorax and abdomen and shows that for this structure the discrepancy is only marginal.

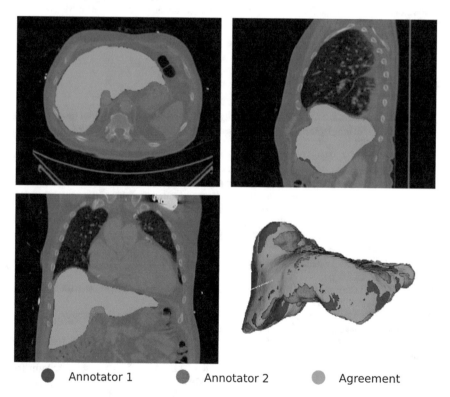

● Annotator 1   ● Annotator 2   ● Agreement

Fig. 4.9 Visualization of the agreement of two annotators based on a liver segmentation in a contrast-enhanced CT volume of the thorax and abdominal region

4.5 Conclusion

This chapter described the annotation of medical images that was performed in the VISCERAL project. Both the selection of the tool to annotate the 3D images and the quality management of the annotations are extremely important. A good choice of an annotation tool can significantly limit the amount of work required to do the annotations. Semi-automatic solutions like the ones chosen allow to rapidly achieve good segmentation results.

The quality management also showed that this process can be automated to optimize the outcomes. Not only is a detailed description of the structures to annotate important, but also regular controls and manual checks to compare the written description with the actual practice. There is always subjectivity in annotations, so double annotations are essential to judge the subjectivity of a task. However, only if the control is systematic can the subjectivity be limited and estimated well.

Acknowledgements The research leading to these results has received funding from the European Union Seventh Framework Programme (FP7/2007–2013) under grant agreement 318068 (VISCERAL).

References

1. Bitter I, Van Uitert R, Wolf I, Ibanez L, Kuhnigk JM (2007) Comparison of four freely available frameworks for image processing and visualization that use ITK. IEEE Trans Vis Comput Graph 13(3):483–493
2. Caban JJ, Joshi A, Nagy P (2007) Rapid development of medical imaging tools with open-source libraries. J Digit Imaging 20(1):83–93
3. Chapman BE, Wong M, Farcas C, Reynolds P (2012) Annio: a web-based tool for annotating medical images with ontologies. In: 2012 IEEE second international conference on healthcare informatics, imaging and systems biology. IEEE, New Jersey, p 147
4. Criminisi A, Sharp T, Blake A (2008) GeoS: geodesic image segmentation. In: Forsyth D, Torr P, Zisserman A (eds) ECCV 2008. LNCS, vol 5302. Springer, Heidelberg, pp 99–112. doi:10.1007/978-3-540-88682-2_9
5. Dice LR (1945) Measures of the amount of ecologic association between species. Ecology 26(3):297–302
6. Doi K (2005) Current status and future potential of computer-aided diagnosis in medical imaging. Br J Radiol 78:3–19
7. Engle RL (1992) Attempts to use computers as diagnostic aids in medical decision making: a thirty-year experience. Perspect Biol Med 35(2):207–219
8. Hanbury A, Müller H, Langs G, Weber MA, Menze BH, Fernandez TS (2012) Bringing the algorithms to the data: cloud-based benchmarking for medical image analysis. In: Catarci T, Forner P, Hiemstra D, Peñas A, Santucci G (eds) CLEF 2012. LNCS, vol 7488. Springer, Heidelberg, pp 24–29. doi:10.1007/978-3-642-33247-0_3
9. Langs G, Hanbury A, Menze B, Müller H (2013) VISCERAL: towards large data in medical imaging — challenges and directions. In: Greenspan H, Müller H, Syeda-Mahmood T (eds) MCBR-CDS 2012. LNCS, vol 7723. Springer, Heidelberg, pp 92–98. doi:10.1007/978-3-642-36678-9_9

10. Mata C, Oliver A, Torrent A, Marti J (2012) Mammoapplet: an interactive Java applet tool for manual annotation in medical imaging. In: 2012 IEEE 12th international conference on bioinformatics and bioengineering (BIBE). IEEE, New Jersey, pp 34–39
11. Pieper S, Halle M, Kikinis R (2004) 3D slicer. In: IEEE international symposium on biomedical imaging: nano to macro. IEEE, New Jersey, pp 632–635
12. Sharma N, Aggarwal LM (2010) Automated medical image segmentation techniques. J Med Phys Assoc Med Phys India 35(1):3
13. Jiménez-del Toro OA, Müller H, Krenn M, Gruenberg K, Taha AA, Winterstein M, Eggel I, Foncubierta-Rodríguez A, Goksel O, Jakab A, Kontokotsios G, Langs G, Menze B, Salas Fernandez T, Schaer R, Walleyo A, Weber MA, Dicente Cid Y, Gass T, Heinrich M, Jia F, Kahl F, Kechichian R, Mai D, Spanier AB, Vincent G, Wang C, Wyeth D, Hanbury A (2016) Cloud-based evaluation of anatomical structure segmentation and landmark detection algorithms: visceral anatomy benchmarks. IEEE Trans Med Imaging 35(11):2459–2475
14. Yushkevich PA, Piven J, Hazlett HC, Smith RG, Ho S, Gee JC, Gerig G (2006) User-guided 3D active contour segmentation of anatomical structures: significantly improved efficiency and reliability. Neuroimage 31(3):1116–1128
15. Zou KH, Warfield SK, Bharatha A, Tempany CM, Kaus MR, Haker SJ, Wells WM III, Jolesz FA, Kikinis R (2004) Statistical validation of image segmentation quality based on a spatial overlap index[1]: scientific reports. Acad Radiol 11(2):178–189

Chapter 5
Datasets Created in VISCERAL

**Markus Krenn, Katharina Grünberg, Oscar Jimenez-del-Toro,
András Jakab, Tomàs Salas Fernandez, Marianne Winterstein,
Marc-André Weber and Georg Langs**

Abstract In the VISCERAL project, several *Gold Corpus* datasets containing medical imaging data and corresponding manual expert annotations have been created. These datasets were used for training and evaluation of participant algorithms in the VISCERAL Benchmarks. In addition to Gold Corpus datasets, the architecture of VISCERAL enables the creation of *Silver Corpus* annotations of far larger datasets, which are generated by the collective ensemble of submitted algorithms. In this chapter, three Gold Corpus datasets created for the VISCERAL Anatomy, Detection and Retrieval Benchmarks are described. Additionally, we present two datasets that have been created as a result of the anatomy and retrieval challenge.

Source code is available at:
https://github.com/Visceral-Project/silverCorpusFramework

M. Krenn (✉) · G. Langs · A. Jakab
Medical University of Vienna, Spitalgasse 23, 1090 Vienna, Austria
e-mail: markus.krenn@meduniwien.ac.at; max@contentflow.com

G. Langs
e-mail: georg.langs@meduniwien.ac.at

K. Grünberg · M. Winterstein · M.-A. Weber
University of Heidelberg, Heidelberg, Germany
e-mail: katharina.gruenberg@med.uni-heidelberg.de

T. Salas Fernandez
Agencia D'Informació, Avaluació I Qualitat En Salut, Barcelona, Spain

O. Jimenez-del-Toro
University of Applied Sciences Western Switzerland, Sierre, Switzerland
e-mail: oscar.jimenez@hevs.ch

© The Author(s) 2017
A. Hanbury et al. (eds.), *Cloud-Based Benchmarking
of Medical Image Analysis*, DOI 10.1007/978-3-319-49644-3_5

5.1 Introduction

One of the main objectives of the VISCERAL project has been to provide substantial Gold Corpus datasets to the medical image analysis research community containing medical imaging data complemented with manual annotations performed by experienced radiologists. For each benchmark organized within the project, a Gold Corpus dataset was created in order to train and evaluate the participants' algorithms.

In addition to the Gold Corpus of expert-annotated imaging data, the architecture of the VISCERAL Benchmarks offers the possibility to generate far larger Silver Corpus data that are annotated by the collective ensemble of algorithms submitted by Benchmark participants. Even though these Silver Corpus annotations are expected to be less accurate than Gold Corpus annotations, we encourage the idea of their creation since they can be generated automatically and therefore created on larger scales than is feasible to achieve with expert annotations. Furthermore, experiments showed that the pooling of algorithm results did provide enhanced annotations over individual algorithms [1].

The following sections describe Gold Corpus and Silver Corpus datasets created as part of VISCERAL.

5.2 Anatomy Gold Corpus

The Anatomy Gold Corpus was created to provide substantial training and test data for the Anatomy Benchmarks 1–3, in which participants have been challenged with the tasks of labelling anatomical structures (segmentation) on the one hand and detecting landmarks (localization) in medical imaging data on the other hand.

The dataset contains 120 3D medical images (volumes) acquired during daily clinical routine and cover four different imaging modalities. Table 5.1 lists and describes the modalities, their fields of view and voxel dimensions.

Each volume carries two types of anatomical reference annotations performed by experienced radiologists that serve as gold standard references:

Table 5.1 Imaging modalities covered by the VISCERAL Anatomy Gold Corpus

Identifier	Modality	Field of view	Voxel dimensions (in mm)
CT-Wb	CT	whole body	$0.8 - 0.9 \times 0.8 - 0.9 \times 1.5$
CTce-ThAb	contrast-enhanced CT	thorax and abdomen	$0.6 - 0.7 \times 0.6 - 0.7 \times 1.2 - 1.5$
MRT1-Wb	MRI - T1 weighted	whole body	$1.1 - 1.3 \times 1.1 - 1.3 \times 6 - 7$
MRT1cefs-Ab	contrast-enhanced fat-saturated MRI - T1 weighted	abdomen	$1.2 - 1.3 \times 1.2 - 1.3 \times 3$

Table 5.2 Overview of the VISCERAL Anatomy Gold Corpus

Category	# Volumes	# Structures	# Landmarks
CT-Wb	30	573	1574
CTce-ThAb	30	583	1244
MRT1-Wb	30	442	1447
MRT1-ThAb	30	322	595
$\sum$	**120**	**1920**	**4860**

1. **Segmentation labels**: A labelling of up to 20 anatomical structures such as kidneys, lungs, liver, urinary bladder, pancreas, adrenal glands, thyroid glands, aorta and some muscles.
2. **Landmark labels**: Up to 53 anatomical landmarks including the lateral end of the clavicula, crista iliaca, symphysis, trochanter major/minor, tip of aortic arch, trachea/aortic bifurcation, crista iliaca and the vertebrae.

An anatomical structure annotation is given in the form of a 3D image, where the value 0 in a voxel indicates absence (background) and a value > 0 indicates presence (foreground) of a specific structure. All annotated landmarks of an image are given as a list where an entry holds the landmark name and its x-, y- and z- coordinates.

In VISCERAL, the Neuroimaging Informatics Technology Initiative (NIfTI)[1] file format is used to store medical imaging data. In contrast to the slice-based Digital Imaging and Communications in Medicine (DICOM)[2] standard, the full volume is stored as a single self-contained file. This facilitates file management considerably, since transfer and storage of thousands of large files instead of millions of small files are typically more efficient.

Table 5.2 lists the number of volumes, annotated structures and landmarks that build the VISCERAL Anatomy Gold Corpus. Overall, 30 volumes of each modality have been annotated, resulting in a dataset that consists of 120 volumes with 1920 corresponding structures and 4860 landmark annotations. Detailed breakdowns of annotations per structure and landmark in each modality are given in Tables 5.3 and 5.4, where Table 5.3 provides a breakdown of manually annotated anatomical structures per modality in volumes of the Anatomy Gold Corpus dataset, and Table 5.4 lists landmark annotations that have been annotated by radiology experts and are available in volumes of the Gold Corpus. Missing annotations are due to poor visibility of the structures in certain image modalities or due to such structures being outside of the field of view. Figure 5.1 illustrates Gold Corpus annotations in one volume of each modality.

---

[1] Neuroimaging Informatics Technology Initiative: http://nifti.nimh.nih.gov/.
[2] Digital Imaging and Communications in Medicine: http://dicom.nema.org/.

Table 5.3 Manual annotations of anatomical structures performed by experienced radiologists available in the Anatomy Gold Corpus

Structure	CT-Wb	Ctce-ThAb	MRT1-Wb	MRT1cefs-Ab	$\sum$
Adrenal gland (L)	24	28	17	16	**85**
Adrenal gland (R)	21	28	14	8	**71**
Aorta	30	30	30	10	**100**
First lumbar vertebra	30	30	29	22	**111**
Gallbladder	25	29	9	14	**77**
Kidney (L)	29	30	30	28	**117**
Kidney (R)	30	30	30	28	**118**
Liver	30	30	28	30	**118**
Lung (L)	30	30	30	7	**97**
Lung (R)	30	30	30	7	**97**
M. b. rectus abdominis (L)	30	30	4	7	**71**
M. b. rectus abdominis (R)	30	30	4	6	**70**
Pancreas	30	28	9	21	**88**
Psoas major (L)	30	30	30	29	**119**
Psoas major (R)	30	30	30	30	**120**
Spleen	30	30	30	29	**119**
Sternum	30	30	7		**67**
Thyroid gland	25	20	21		**66**
Trachea	30	30	30		**90**
Urinary bladder	29	30	30	30	**119**
$\sum$	573	583	442	322	1920

Table 5.4 Annotated landmarks per modality available in volumes of the Anatomy Gold Corpus

Landmark	CT-Wb	Ctce-ThAb	MRT1-Wb	MRT1cefs-Ab	$\sum$
Aorta bifurcation	30	30	29	30	**119**
Aortic arch	30	30	29	2	**91**
Aortic valve	29	30	24		**83**
Bronchus (L)	30	28	25		**83**
Bronchus (R)	30	28	27		**85**
C2	28		29		**57**
C3	29		29		**58**
C4	29		29		**58**
C5	29		29		**58**
C6	29	6	29		**64**
C7	29	22	29		**80**
Clavicle (L)	30	13	30	30	**103**
Clavicle (R)	30	13	30	30	**103**

(continued)

Table 5.4   (continued)

Landmark	CT-Wb	Ctce-ThAb	MRT1-Wb	MRT1cefs-Ab	Σ
Coronaria	23	22	1		46
Crista iliaca (L)	30	30	30		90
Crista iliaca (R)	30	30	30		90
Eye (L)	30		5		35
Eye (R)	30		5		35
Ischiadicum (L)	30	30	29	24	113
Ischiadicum (R)	30	30	29	24	113
L1	30	30	30	30	120
L2	30	30	30	30	120
L3	30	30	30	30	120
L4	30	31	30	30	121
L5	30	30	30	30	120
Renalpelvis (L)	29	30	29	27	115
Renalpelvis (R)	30	30	30	27	117
Sternoclavicular (L)	30	30	27		87
Sternoclavicular (R)	30	30	27		87
Symphysis	30	30	29	30	119
Th1	30	30	30		90
Th2	30	30	31		91
Th3	30	30	28		88
Th4	30	30	29		89
Th5	30	30	29		89
Th6	30	30	29	1	90
Th7	30	30	30	3	93
Th8	30	30	30	5	95
Th9	30	30	30	9	99
Th10	30	30	30	19	109
Th11	30	30	30	25	115
Th12	30	30	29	28	117
Trachea bifurcation	30	29	29		88
Trochanter major (L)	30	30	30	22	112
Trochanter major (R)	30	30	30	24	114
Trochanter minor (L)	30	29	30	20	109
Trochanter minor (R)	30	29	30	20	109
Tuberculum (L)	30	17	30		77
Tuberculum (R)	30	17	30		77
Vci bifurcation	30	30	27		87
Ventricle (L)	30		29		59
Ventricle (R)	30		29	30	89
Xyphoideus	30	30	9	15	84
Σ	1574	1244	1447	595	4860

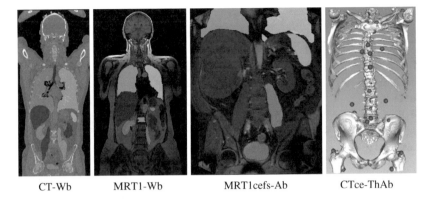

CT-Wb   MRT1-Wb   MRT1cefs-Ab   CTce-ThAb

Fig. 5.1 Anatomical structure annotations in CT, MRT1 and a MRT1cefs volume *(a-c)* and visualization of annotated landmarks in a CTce volume *(d)*

5.3 Anatomy Silver Corpus

The Anatomy Silver Corpus was created based on the data and results available from the segmentation tasks of Anatomy 2 and 3 Benchmarks [2, 3]. Here, segmentations of all organs addressed within the benchmark were created by fusing multiple segmentation estimates originating from (1) the submitted algorithms and (2) Gold Corpus annotations transformed by medical image registration methods. The process to derive a Silver Corpus annotation of a specific structure in a novel volume is described and discussed in detail in [1] and can be summarized as follows:

1. Compute algorithmic segmentation estimates by applying all submitted algorithms to the target image.
2. Transfer manual annotations of Gold Corpus volumes to the target image by a preregistration selection, image registration and label propagation approach.
3. Build consensus of all segmentation estimates (algorithmic and atlas based) using the SIMPLE [4] segmentation approach.

This procedure has been applied to 264 additional volumes of the modalities covered by the Gold Corpus, resulting in up to 20 automatically generated Silver

Table 5.5 Overview of the VISCERAL Anatomy Silver Corpus dataset

Category	# Volumes	# Structures	# Landmarks
CT-Wb	62	1122	3169
CTce-ThAb	65	1227	2600
MRT1-Wb	66	1095	3136
MRT1-ThAb	71	879	1342
$\sum$	**264**	**4323**	**10247**

Table 5.6 Segmentation accuracy (μ, σ) of the silver corpus fusion process evaluated on 10 volumes of the Gold Corpus per modality and number of Silver Corpus annotations (#) computed on additional volumes that are available as a resource for the research community

Anatomical structure	CT			CTce			MRT1			MRT1cefs		
	#	μ	σ	#	μ	σ	#	μ	σ	#	μ	σ
Adrenal gland (L)	54	0.36	0.19	53	0.35	0.17	41	0.17	0.22	49	0.21	0.12
Adrenal gland (R)	54	0.32	0.2	56	0.35	0.14	50	0.38	0.14	60	0.23	0.11
Aorta	58	0.79	0.04	63	0.82	0.05	65	0.73	0.07	71	0.68	0.02
First lumbar vertebra	57	0.67	0.36	63	0.68	0.34	58	0.46	0.25	71	0.23	0.12
Gallbladder	40	0.24	0.19	49	0.54	0.15	46	0.05	0.05	61	0.13	0.2
Kidney (L)	58	0.9	0.03	63	0.93	0.02	64	0.84	0.06	71	0.85	0.2
Kidney (R)	57	0.87	0.12	63	0.94	0.01	65	0.81	0.11	71	0.86	0.18
Liver	59	0.93	0.01	63	0.94	0.01	66	0.83	0.07	71	0.9	0.03
Lung (L)	61	0.97	0.01	63	0.97	0.01	66	0.91	0.03	-	-	-
Lung (R)	60	0.98	0.01	64	0.97	0.01	66	0.92	0.02	-	-	-
M. b. rectus abdominis (L)	55	0.64	0.14	64	0.63	0.17	-	-	-	-	-	-
M. b. rectus abdominis (R)	56	0.6	0.21	63	0.69	0.16	-	-	-	-	-	-
Pancreas	57	0.43	0.19	60	0.47	0.18	63	0.21	0.21	71	0.46	0.13
Psoas major (L)	56	0.84	0.02	63	0.85	0.05	65	0.82	0.06	71	0.8	0.05
Psoas major (R)	58	0.84	0.02	63	0.86	0.02	65	0.79	0.06	71	0.73	0.12
Spleen	55	0.89	0.06	63	0.89	0.07	65	0.74	0.11	71	0.79	0.18
Sternum	55	0.8	0.04	63	0.83	0.07	64	0.6	0	-	-	-
Thyroid gland	57	0.57	0.1	62	0.52	0.13	64	0.25	0.15	-	-	-
Trachea	57	0.93	0.02	62	0.93	0.02	63	0.78	0.1	-	-	-
Urinary bladder	58	0.76	0.15	64	0.86	0.06	59	0.66	0.28	70	0.45	0.25
Σ	1122			1227			1095			879		

Corpus segmentations per volume. In addition to the segmentation of organs, each volume is complemented with manually performed landmark annotations similar to those of the Gold Corpus. This results in the VISCERAL Anatomy Silver Corpus that contains over 4.000 automatically generated segmentations of anatomical structures and more than 10.000 annotated landmarks.

Table 5.5 outlines the number of volumes, structure segmentations and landmark annotations in each modality available in the Silver Corpus. Detailed breakdowns of segmentations per structure and landmarks for each modality are given in Tables 5.6 and 5.7. Table 5.6 lists the number of computed segmentations (#) per structure and modality together with average segmentation performances (μ) and corresponding standard deviations (σ) of Silver Corpus segmentations computed and compared to Gold Corpus annotations of 40 volumes. These results serve as structure- and modality-specific segmentation performance estimates of generated Silver Corpus annotations. Table 5.7 lists annotated landmarks per modality of the VISCERAL Anatomy Silver Corpus.

For reference, Fig. 5.2 shows average Dice coefficients [5] obtained by comparing Silver Corpus segmentations computed in 10 volumes per modality of the Gold

Table 5.7 Annotated landmarks per modality of the Anatomy Silver Corpus

Landmark	CT-Wb	Ctce-ThAb	MRT1-Wb	MRT1cefs-Ab	Σ
Aorta bifurcation	62	63	64	70	**259**
Aortic arch	51	57	54		**162**
Aortic valve	48	57	34		**139**
Bronchus (L)	62	63	51		**176**
Bronchus (R)	62	63	55		**180**
C2	61	3	65		**129**
C3	62	3	65		**130**
C4	62	3	65		**130**
C5	62	4	65		**131**
C6	62	13	65		**140**
C7	62	52	65		**179**
Clavicle (L)	62	20	65		**147**
Clavicle (R)	62	22	64		**148**
Coronaria	12	36	1		**49**
Crista iliaca (L)	62	61	63	70	**256**
Crista iliaca (R)	62	61	64	70	**257**
Eye (L)	63		23		**86**
Eye (R)	61		23		**84**
Ischiadicum (L)	62	62	65	54	**243**
Ischiadicum (R)	62	62	63	54	**241**

(continued)

Table 5.7   (continued)

Landmark	CT-Wb	Ctce-ThAb	MRT1-Wb	MRT1cefs-Ab	Σ
L1	62	63	65	68	**258**
L2	62	63	65	70	**260**
L3	62	63	64	71	**260**
L4	61	63	65	71	**260**
L5	60	63	63	71	**257**
Renalpelvis (L)	61	62	64	69	**256**
Renalpelvis (R)	61	62	64	66	**253**
Sternoclavicular (L)	62	63	59		**184**
Sternoclavicular (R)	62	63	59		**184**
Symphysis	62	64	64	68	**258**
Th1	62	63	65		**190**
Th2	62	63	65		**190**
Th3	62	64	65		**191**
Th4	62	63	65		**190**
Th5	61	63	65		**189**
Th6	62	63	65		**190**
Th7	62	63	65		**190**
Th8	62	63	65	8	**198**
Th9	62	63	65	15	**205**
Th10	62	63	65	33	**223**
Th11	62	63	65	50	**240**
Th12	62	63	65	60	**250**
Trachea bifurcation	62	62	64		**188**
Trochanter major (L)	62	64	65	60	**251**
Trochanter major (R)	62	64	65	59	**250**
Trochanter minor (L)	61	63	64	52	**240**
Trochanter minor (R)	61	62	64	52	**239**
Tuberculum (L)	61	31	61		**153**
Tuberculum (R)	62	38	63		**163**
Vci bifurcation	60	63	64	65	**252**
Ventricle (L)	48		62		**110**
Ventricle (R)	48		63		**111**
Xyphoideus	60	62	10	16	**148**
Σ	**3169**	**2600**	**3136**	**1342**	**10247**

Corpus to the corresponding manual ground truth annotation. These results can be interpreted as structure and modality-specific segmentation performance estimates of generated Silver Corpus annotations. Average segmentation accuracy (μ) and

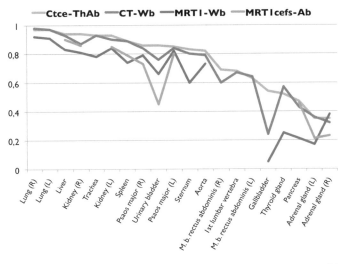

Fig. 5.2 Accuracy (DICE) of Silver Corpus segmentations evaluated on 10 volumes of the Anatomy Gold Corpus

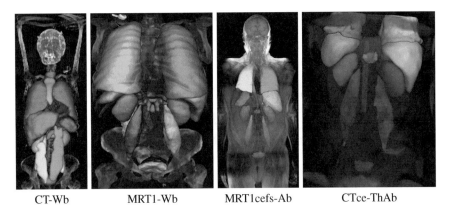

| CT-Wb | MRT1-Wb | MRT1cefs-Ab | CTce-ThAb |

Fig. 5.3 Illustrations of generated Silver Corpus annotations in one volume of each modality. Figures taken from [1]

corresponding standard deviations (σ) are provided in Table 5.6. Figure 5.3 illustrates computed Silver Corpus segmentations in one volume of each modality. The software for creating the Silver Corpus is available.[3]

---

[3]https://github.com/Visceral-Project/silverCorpusFramework.

5.4   Detection Gold Corpus

In the VISCERAL Detection Benchmark, participants have been challenged to develop algorithms that automatically detect and identify lesions in medical imaging data. The Gold Corpus created for test and training purposes in this context thus consists of a set of medical images in which lesions have been manually annotated by the experienced radiologists.

The dataset includes volumes of two modalities (CT-Wb & MRT2-Wb) in which all lesions of five predefined target structures (bones, brain, liver, lung and lymph nodes) have been annotated. A lesion is identified by one point that indicates the centre of a lesion and two additional points on the perimeter to give an estimate of the diameter. Since lesions are not spherical, this is an estimate, but in the context of the Detection Benchmark still is clinically relevant. All lesion annotations of a volume are given in an *fcsv* file containing a list of annotated points and their x-, y- and z-coordinates labelled according to the following naming convention:

structure_counter_identifier, where

- *structure* indicates in which anatomical structure the lesion is located (bones BO, brain BR, liver LI, lungs LU and lymph nodes LN),
- *counter* depicts the index of a lesion within an anatomical structure and
- *identifier* defines if the annotated point represents the centre (C) or diameter estimate (D1, D2) of a specific lesion.

Figure 5.4 gives an example of a lesion annotation file and shows the three points (C, D1 and D2) that represent a bone lesion annotation in a MRT2 image. In total, 1609 lesions have been annotated in 100 volumes. Table 5.8 gives an overview of volumes and lesions annotated per modality and target structure. Example lesion annotations in all target structures of both modalities are shown in Fig. 5.5.

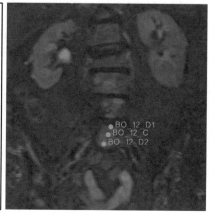

```
# VISCERAL - Detection Benchmark
# Lesion annotation file
#
# Each row contains one point of
# a lesion annotation
# Each lesion has three annotated points:
#  The centre of the lesion (C) and
#  2 points to estimate the diameter (D1,D2)
#
# Each annotation is named according
# to the following convention
#   <targetStructure>_<counter>_<pointIdentifier>
#
# columns = lesionIdentifier,x,y,z
#
#
BO_1_C,118.779,6.168,-657.02
BO_1_D1,118.401,6.168,-651.99
BO_1_D2,117.834,6.168,-663.44
BO_2_C,128.098,18.1587,-698.30
BO_2_D1,128.253,18.1587,-695.20
BO_2_D2,127.633,18.1587,-700.94
```

Fig. 5.4 Example of a lesion annotation file and illustration of an annotated bone lesion

Table 5.8 Number of volumes and lesions annotated in the VISCERAL detection Gold Corpus

Modality	# Volumes	# Annotated lesions					$\sum$
		Bone	Lungs	Liver	Lymph nodes	Brain	
CT - WB	50	911	24	27	48	2	1012
MRT2 - WB	50	541	5	44	1	6	597
$\sum$	**100**	**1452**	**29**	**71**	**49**	**8**	**1609**

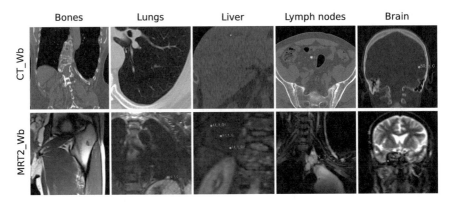

Fig. 5.5 Exemplary lesion annotations in all target structures of both modalities annotated

5.5 Retrieval Gold Corpus

Participants of the VISCERAL Retrieval Benchmark were challenged to find clinically relevant or similar cases to a given query case in a large multimodal dataset. For this purpose, a Gold Corpus has been created that contains:

1. Medical images from multiple modalities, covering different parts of the human body.
2. Anatomy–Pathology (AP) terms exported from corresponding radiology reports that describe which pathological findings occur in which anatomical regions of an image.

Annotations of findings in an image are given in the form of AP term files that list terms describing pathologies that occur in the radiology report of an image together with its anatomy. Both entities are described textually and with their corresponding RadLex ID[4] (RID). RadLex is a unified terminology of radiology terms that can be used for standardized indexing and retrieval of radiology information resources. AP term files furthermore indicate whether a pathology has been explicitly negated in the report. Figure 5.6 shows an example of an AP term file. This file indicates for instance

---

[4]http://rsna.org/RadLex.aspx.

```
VolumeID_Modality_Bodyregion.fcsv
i.e. 123456_MRT1_Ab.csv
```
```
# The first row depicts the header of an a-p term file.
Anatomy RID,Anatomy,Pathology RID,Pathology,Negated
#
# Each row entry in this file contains an occurring pathology and its anatomy and
states if the pathology is negated.
RID199,Ductus choledochus,RID4865,Ödem,1
RID58,Leber,RID3874,Raumforderung,0
```

Fig. 5.6 Example of an AP term file

Table 5.9 Number of volumes and available AP term files of the VISCERAL retrieval Gold Corpus

Modality	Field of view	# Volumes	# AP term files
CT	Abdomen	336	213
	Thorax & Abdomen	86	86
	Thorax	971	699
	Unknown	211	211
	Whole body	410	410
MRT1	Abdomen	167	114
	Unknown	24	24
MRT2	Abdomen	68	18
	Unknown	38	38
Σ		**2311**	**1813**

that volume *123456_MRT1_Ab* does not contain the pathological finding *Oedem* in *Ductus choledochus* but contains *Raumforderung* in the anatomical structure *Leber*.

The dataset consists of 2311 volumes originated from three different modalities (CT, MRT1, and MRT2) which have been acquired during clinical routine. For 1813 cases of the dataset, AP term files are available and thus part of the retrieval Gold Corpus. Table 5.9 gives a detailed overview of the number of volumes per modality and field of view and lists available AP term files that form the VISCERAL Retrieval Gold Corpus.

5.6   Retrieval Silver Corpus

Participants of the VISCERAL Retrieval Benchmark have been challenged to find clinically relevant cases in the Retrieval Gold Corpus for given queries. For this purpose, ten query cases (illustrated in Fig. 5.7) have been created, where each query in this scenario has been defined by:

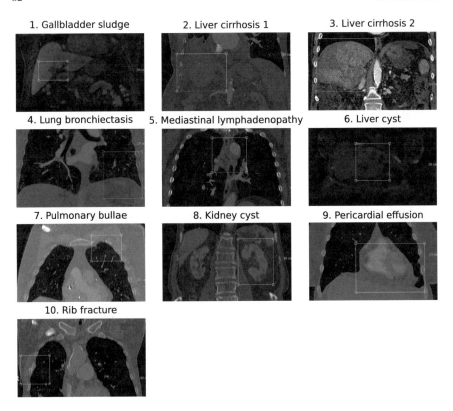

Fig. 5.7 Illustration of the query cases of the Detection Benchmark

- The AP term that defines the topic of a query, i.e. liver – cyst,
- The 3D medical image data (CT, MRT1 and MRT2),
- A 3D bounding box of the region that contains radiological signs of the pathology,
- A binary mask of the organ affected and
- The AP term list extracted from the volumes report.

During evaluation, medical experts performed relevance judgements of the top-ranked cases submitted to each query to judge the quality of retrieval of each participant's approach. This process results in a set of clinically relevant and irrelevant cases from the Gold Corpus for each given query, which builds the VISCERAL Retrieval Silver Corpus.

In total, 6240 relevance judgements have been performed in this context from which 2462 cases are clinically relevant and 3778 are not relevant to one of the given queries. Table 5.10 shows the corresponding numbers of relevant and not relevant cases of the Gold Corpus for each query.

Table 5.10 Retrieval Silver Corpus. Number of clinically relevant and not relevant cases of the Gold Corpus for each query

Query	Relevant	Not relevant	$\sum$
Gallbladder sludge	118	194	312
Liver cirrhosis 1	428	395	823
Liver cirrhosis 2	428	395	823
Lung bronchiectasis	161	453	614
Mediastinal lymphadenopathy	248	342	590
Liver cyst	339	264	603
Pulmonary bullae	333	258	591
Kidney cyst	336	263	599
Pericardial effusion	24	696	720
Rib fracture	47	518	565
$\sum$	**2462**	**3778**	**6240**

5.7 Summary

During the VISCERAL project, we have generated datasets of medical imaging data together with annotations. The purpose of the VISCERAL Gold Corpora is to serve as training set for algorithm development and for evaluation of algorithms. The VISCERAL Silver Corpora use the results of algorithms to create algorithmic annotations on far larger datasets.

Three so-called *Gold Corpus* datasets have been created containing medical imaging data and corresponding gold standard annotations:

1. The **VISCERAL Anatomy Gold Corpus** consists of 120 medical images of four modalities and carries (1) 1920 voxel-wise annotations of up to 20 anatomical structures per volume and (2) 4860 annotated landmarks of up to 53 predefined points of interest per volume.
2. The **VISCERAL Detection Gold Corpus** contains 100 medical images of two modalities and provides annotations of 1609 lesions in five anatomies (bones, lungs, liver lymph nodes and brain).
3. The **VISCERAL Retrieval Gold Corpus** includes 2311 medical images of three modalities, where for 1813 cases the corresponding radiology report-extracted AP terms are available that describe occurring pathological findings and their anatomy.

Furthermore, two *Silver Corpus* datasets have been generated based on the data and results available from Anatomy and Retrieval Benchmarks:

1. The **VISCERAL Anatomy Silver Corpus** provides automatically generated silver standard segmentations of up to 20 anatomical structures in 264 volumes (4323 in total) and additionally manual landmark annotations in each of these volumes (>10.000 annotations).

2. The **VISCERAL Retrieval Silver Corpus** provides a list of relevant and irrelevant cases of the Retrieval Gold Corpus to each query case of the Retrieval Benchmark.

Acknowledgements The research leading to these results has received funding from the European Union Seventh Framework Programme (FP7/2007–2013) under grant agreement 318068 (VISCERAL).

References

1. Krenn M, Dorfer M, Jiménez del Toro OA, Müller H, Menze B, Weber MA, Hanbury A, Langs G (2016) Creating a large-scale silver corpus from multiple algorithmic segmentations. In: Menze B, Langs G, Montillo A, Kelm M, Müller H, Zhang S, Cai W, Metaxas D (eds) MCV 2015. LNCS, vol 9601. Springer, Cham, pp 103–115. doi:10.1007/978-3-319-42016-5_10
2. Göksel O, Jiménez-del Toro OA, Foncubierta-Rodríguez A, Müller H (2015) Overview of the visceral challenge at ISBI 2015. In: Proceedings of the VISCERAL challenge at ISBI, New York
3. Jiménez del Toro O, Goksel O, Menze B, Müller H, Langs G, Weber M, Eggel I, Gruenberg K, Holzer M, Jakab A, Kotsios-Kontokotsios G, Krenn M, Salas Fernandez T, Schaer R, Taha AA, Winterstein M, Hanbury A (2014) Visceral—visual concept extraction challenge in radiology: ISBI 2014 challenge organization. In: Göksel O (ed) Proceedings of the VISCERAL challenge at ISBI, CEUR workshop proceedings, pp 6–15
4. Langerak TR, van der Heide UA, Kotte ANTJ, Viergever MA, van Vulpen M, Pluim JPW (2010) Label fusion in atlas-based segmentation using a selective and iterative method for performance level estimation (simple). IEEE Trans Med Imaging 29(12):2000–2008
5. Dice LR (1945) Measures of the amount of ecologic association between species. Ecology 26(3):297–302

Part III
VISCERAL Benchmarks

Chapter 6
Evaluation Metrics for Medical Organ Segmentation and Lesion Detection

Abdel Aziz Taha and Allan Hanbury

Abstract This chapter provides an overview of the metrics used in the VISCERAL segmentation benchmarks, namely Anatomy 1, 2 and 3. In particular, it provides an overview of 20 evaluation metrics for segmentation, from which four metrics were selected to be used in VISCERAL benchmarks. It also provides an analysis of these metrics in three ways: first by analysing fuzzy implementations of these metrics using fuzzy segmentations produced either synthetically or by fusing participant segmentations and second by comparing segmentation rankings produced by these metrics with rankings performed manually by radiologists. Finally, a metric selection is performed using an automatic selection framework, and the selection result is validated using the manual rankings. Furthermore, this chapter provides an overview of metrics used for the Lesion Detection Benchmark.

Source code is available at:
https://github.com/visceral-project/EvaluateSegmentation

6.1 Introduction

The importance of using suitable metrics in evaluation stems from the fact that there are different metrics, and each of them has particular sensitivities and thus measures particular aspects of similarity/discrepancy between the objects being evaluated and the corresponding ground truth. Poorly defined metrics may lead to inaccurate conclusions about the state-of-the-art algorithms, which negatively impacts system

A.A. Taha · A. Hanbury (✉)
Institute of Software Technology and Interactive Systems, TU Wien,
Favoritenstraße 9-11/188, 1040 Vienna, Austria
e-mail: hanbury@ifs.tuwien.ac.at

A.A. Taha
e-mail: taha@ifs.tuwien.ac.at

© The Author(s) 2017
A. Hanbury et al. (eds.), *Cloud-Based Benchmarking
of Medical Image Analysis*, DOI 10.1007/978-3-319-49644-3_6

development. This chapter provides an overview of metrics used for the Anatomy and Detection Benchmarks of the VISCERAL project [1].

Segmentation methods with high accuracy and high reproducibility are a main goal in medical image processing. Therefore, assessing the accuracy and the quality of segmentation algorithms is of great importance, which is a matter of the evaluation methodology. Segmentation evaluation is the task of comparing two segmentations by measuring the distance or similarity between them, where one is the segmentation to be evaluated and the other is the corresponding ground truth segmentation. In this chapter, we provide an overview of a metric pool consisting of twenty metrics for evaluating medical image segmentations and a subset of four metrics that were considered in the VISCERAL segmentation benchmarks.

The knowledge about the metrics in terms of their strength, weakness, sensitivities, bias, as well as their ability to deal with fuzzy segmentation, is essential for taking the decision about which metrics are to be used in the evaluation. In this chapter, we provide an analysis of metrics with respect to their fuzzy definitions and discussion about selecting suitable metrics for evaluating segmentation from a metric pool.

Apart from segmentation, the VISCERAL project had also the Lesion Detection Benchmark, where lesions are to be localized by detection algorithms. In this chapter, we provide an overview of the metrics and evaluation methodologies that were used for the Detection Benchmark.

The remainder of this chapter is organized as follows: in Sect. 6.2, we provide an overview of the metrics that were used in the VISCERAL Anatomy and Detection Benchmarks. In Sect. 6.3, we validate a subset of the segmentations of the Anatomy 2 Benchmark against synthetic fuzzy variants of the ground truth and discuss the results. In Sect. 6.4, we present an analysis based on the comparison between rankings produced by the segmentation metrics and manual rankings made by radiologists. Finally, this chapter is concluded in Sect. 6.5.

6.2 Metrics for VISCERAL Benchmarks

In this section, we provide an overview of the metrics that were used in the VISCERAL benchmarks. In particular, we provide a pool of metrics for evaluating medical image segmentation, from which four metrics were selected for the VISCERAL Anatomy Benchmarks. Furthermore, we provide an overview of metrics that were used for the Detection Benchmark.

6.2.1 Metrics for Segmentation

Medical image segmentation assigns each voxel of a medical image to a class, e.g. an anatomical structure. While this assignment is crisp in binary segmentation, it takes

Table 6.1 Overview of evaluation metrics for 3D image segmentation. The symbols in the second column are used to denote the metrics throughout the chapter. The column "category" assigns each metric to one of the categories above. The column "Fuzzy" indicates whether a fuzzy implementation of the metric is available

Metric	Symbol	Category	Fuzzy
Dice coefficient	DICE	Spatial overlap based	yes
Jaccard index	JAC	Spatial overlap based	yes
True-positive rate (sensitivity, recall)	TPR	Spatial overlap based	yes
True-negative rate (specificity)	TNR	Spatial overlap based	yes
False-positive rate (= 1-specificity, fallout)	FPR	Spatial overlap based	yes
False-negative rate (= 1-sensitivity)	FNR	Spatial overlap based	yes
F-measure (F1-measure = Dice)	FMS	Spatial overlap based	yes
Global consistency error	GCE	Spatial overlap based	no
Volumetric similarity	VS	Volume based	yes
Rand index	RI	Pair counting based	yes
Adjusted Rand index	ARI	Pair counting based	yes
Mutual information	MI	Information theoretic based	yes
Variation of information	VOI	Information theoretic based	yes
Interclass correlation	ICC	Probabilistic based	no
Probabilistic distance	PBD	Probabilistic based	yes
Cohen's kappa	KAP	Probabilistic based	yes
Area under ROC curve	AUC	Probabilistic based	yes
Hausdorff distance	HD	Spatial distance based	no
Average distance	AVD	Spatial distance based	no
Mahalanobis distance	MHD	Spatial distance based	no

other forms in fuzzy segmentation, e.g. the degree of membership or the probability that a particular voxel belongs to a particular class. An automatic segmentation is validated by comparing it with the corresponding ground truth segmentation using an evaluation metric.

We describe the metrics for validating medical segmentation in Table 6.1, which were selected based on a literature review of papers in which medical volume segmentations are evaluated. Only metrics with at least two references (papers) of use are considered. These metrics were implemented in the EvaluateSegmentation[1] tool for evaluating medical image segmentation. Taha and Hanbury [4] provide definitions and a comprehensive analysis of these metrics as well as guidelines for metric selection based on the properties of the segmentations being evaluated and the segmentation goal.

---

[1]EvaluateSegmentation is open source software for evaluating medical image segmentation available at https://github.com/visceral-project/EvaluateSegmentation.

Based on the relations between the metrics, their nature and their definition, we group them into six categories, namely:

- **Spatial overlap based (Category 1)**: These are metrics defined based on the spatial overlap between the two segmentations being compared, namely the four basic overlap cardinalities—true positives (TP), true negatives (TN), false positives (FP) and false negatives (FN).
- **Volume based (Category 2)**: Metrics from this category are based on comparing the volume of the segmented region, i.e. they aim to measure the number of voxels segmented compared with the number of voxels in the true segmentation (ground truth).
- **Pair counting based (Category 3)**: Metrics from this category are based on $\binom{n}{2}$ tuples that represent all possible voxel pairs in the image. These tuples can be grouped into four categories depending on where the voxels of each pair are placed according to each of the segmentations being compared. These four groups are Group I: if both voxels are placed in the same segment in both segmentations; Group II: if both voxels are placed in the same segment in the first segmentation but in different segments in the second; Group III: if both voxels are placed in the same segment in the second segmentation but in different segments in the first; and Group IV: if both voxels are placed in different segments in both segmentations.
- **Information theoretic based (Category 4)**: Metrics of this category are based on basic values of information theory such as entropy and mutual information.
- **Probabilistic based (Category 5)**: These metrics consider the segmentations being compared as two distributions. Under this consideration, the metrics are defined based on the classic comparison methods of statistics of these distributions.
- **Spatial distance based (Category 6)**: These metrics aim to summarize distances between all pairs of voxels in the two segmentations being compared, i.e. they provide a one-value measure that represents all pairwise distances.

The aim of this grouping is to enable a reasonable selection when a subset of metrics is to be used, i.e. selecting metrics from different groups to avoid biased results.

For the evaluation of medical image segmentation in the VISCERAL Anatomy Benchmarks, four metrics were selected from the 20 metrics presented in Table 6.1. The following criteria were considered:

- The metrics were selected so that they cover as many different categories as possible from those categories described above.
- From those metrics that meet the criteria above, metrics were selected that have the highest correlation with the rest of the metrics in each category.

Based on these criteria, the following metrics were considered for validating segmentations in all the segmentation benchmarks of the VISCERAL project: the Dice coefficient (DICE), the average distance (AVD), the interclass correlation (ICC) and the adjusted Rand index (ARI).

6.2.2 Metrics for Lesion Detection

The Detection Benchmark considered pathology instead of anatomy. The goal of the benchmark is to automatically detect lesions in images acquired in clinical routine.

In the Detection Benchmark, an annotated lesion, L_i, is represented by three points, namely the centre of the lesion, C_i, and two other points, $D1_i$ and $D2_i$, indicating the diameter of the lesion. Participating algorithms are expected to provide per lesion exactly one point, P_i, as near as possible to the centre of the lesion, C_i.

As mentioned above, it is expected that exactly one point per lesion is retrieved by each participating algorithm. To penalize algorithms that may try to improve the evaluation results by providing many points per lesion, all other points retrieved are considered as false positives. However, annotators have looked at specific regions of the volume, which means that one cannot be sure that other regions are free of lesions. In other words, participating algorithms could detect lesions that were not annotated. To avoid penalizing such lesions, binary masks are used for each volume, which mask only those regions that were manually annotated. Retrieved points that lie outside the mask are not considered in the confusion matrix.

The evaluation of the Detection Benchmark takes place at three different levels:

1. Lesion level: For each annotated lesion, two values are measured, namely

   - Minimum Euclidean distance, $min(d_i)$: For each annotated lesion, the distance to the nearest point retrieved by the participating algorithm is measured as shown in Fig. 6.1. This distance is provided for each annotated lesion, regardless of whether the lesion is considered as detected or not.
   - Detection: A lesion is considered as detected if the point P_i, provided by the algorithm, is within the sphere centred on C_i and has the diameter given by the points $D1_i$ and $D2_i$. In particular, a radius of the sphere, r, is considered, which is equal to the distance between the centre C_i and the farthest of the points $D1_i$ and $D2_i$. That is, a lesion is detected iff $min(d) < r$. In Fig. 6.1, the lesion is detected by the point $P1_i$, but not by $P2_i$.

Fig. 6.1 Schematic representation of a lesion annotated by the centre C_i and the two diameter points $D1_i$ and $D2_i$. The points $P1_i$ and $P2_i$ are retrieved by participating algorithms. $P1_i$ lies within the detection sphere and is thus considered as detected in contrast to the point $P2_i$

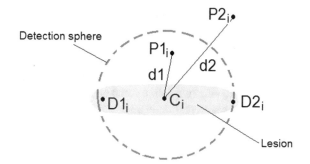

2. Volume level: The confusion matrix (true positives, false positives, true negatives and false negatives) is calculated per volume, based on the detection values calculated at lesion level. From this confusion matrix, the precision (percentage of correctly detected lesions) and the recall (percentage of total lesions detected) are calculated for each volume and participating algorithm. As it is expected that algorithms provide exactly one point per lesion, all further points provided by an algorithm for the same lesion are considered as false positives.
3. Anatomical structure (organ) average level: To test whether the scores of lesion detection are generally dependent on the anatomical structure in which the lesions are, we calculate the score averages (the averages of the Euclidean distances between lesion centres and detection points) over each organ.

6.3   Analysis of Fuzzy Segmentation Metrics

Sometimes, medical volume segmentations are fuzzy. Such segmentations can be the result of averaging annotations done by different annotators. Fuzzy segmentation can also be the result of fusing automatic segmentations, which results in a silver corpus [2]. Depending on the approach used, automatic segmentations generated by segmentation algorithms can also be fuzzy. In contrast to binary segmentation, fuzzy segmentations are represented as memberships of voxels in classes (anatomical structures). Instead of a binary association, a voxel is rather associated with a class with a probability specifying the degree of membership to this class. Note that binary segmentation is just a special case of fuzzy segmentation, where the degree of memberships to a particular class can be either zero or one.

In this section, we analyse the impact of using fuzzy metrics in evaluating medical image segmentation. This is done by analysing the rankings produced by binary and fuzzy metrics of segmentations as well as segmentation algorithms. Segmentation ranking here means ordering segmentations according to their similarities to their corresponding ground truth segmentations. We analyse this from several sides trying to answer the following questions: (1) considering the case when the segmentations being evaluated/ranked are of mixed types (fuzzy and binary), which of the following two evaluation methods is to be used: (a) evaluating both types using fuzzy metrics based on the fact that binary segmentation is a special case of fuzzy segmentation, or (b) cutting fuzzy segmentations at a particular threshold and then using binary evaluation metrics? (2) The same question holds for the case when the ground truth segmentations and the segmentations being evaluated are of different types?

In the following, we define some notations and settings to be used in this section. Since binary segmentation is a special case of fuzzy segmentation, in which probabilities are either 0 or 1, this implies that fuzzy metrics can be used to compare the following combinations of segmentations, which we will denote as evaluation cases throughout this section:

Case i: binary segmentation evaluated against binary ground truth
Case ii: binary segmentation evaluated against fuzzy ground truth

Case iii: fuzzy segmentation evaluated against binary ground truth
Case iv: fuzzy segmentation evaluated against fuzzy ground truth

We define two types of evaluation that can be used for each of the evaluation cases above. The first type is **threshold evaluation**. Here, the ground truth segmentation, as well as the segmentation being evaluated, is cut at a threshold of 0.5 as a first step and then compared using an evaluation metric. The second type is **fuzzy evaluation** in which the segmentations are compared directly using fuzzy metrics.

The aim of this analysis is to infer how sensitive metrics are against image fuzzi-fication. This analysis is motivated by the following: on the one hand, if there is fuzzy ground truth available and the segmentations being evaluated are fuzzy as well (Case iv), then metrics with high fuzzification sensitivity are required to distinguish the accuracy of the systems. On the other hand, when binary segmentations are to be compared with fuzzy ones (Case ii and Case iii), the question to be answered is, which type of evaluation (threshold evaluation or fuzzy evaluation) should be used?

In the Anatomy 1 and 2 Benchmarks, only binary ground truth segmentation has been used. Most of the participating algorithms provided binary segmentation, i.e. from Case i. However, only one of the participating algorithms produced fuzzy segmentations, i.e. Case iii. This algorithm is denoted as *Algorithm A* throughout this section. To complete the analysis, the other cases (Case ii and Case iv) and different types of segmentations are involved, which are described in the following:

- Binary ground truth (BGT): This is the official binary ground truth, used for vali-dating the challenge.
- Synthetic fuzzy ground truth (FGT): Since there are only binary ground truth segmentations available, the fuzzy ground truth was generated synthetically: from each of the ground truth segmentations, a fuzzy variant was produced by smoothing the corresponding ground truth using a mean filter.
- Fuzzy silver ground truth (FSGT): In another variant, a fuzzy silver corpus is generated by fusing all the automatic segmentations.
- Binary silver ground truth (BSGT) [2]: The silver corpus was generated by fusing all the automatic segmentations and then cutting them at threshold 0.5, i.e. BSGT is FSGT cut at 0.5.
- Fuzzy automatic segmentation (FAS): These are the fuzzy segmentations produced by one of the participating algorithms, namely Algorithm A.
- Binary automatic segmentations (BAS): These are the automatic segmentations produced by all of the participating algorithms except Algorithm A.

Metrics considered in this analysis are those metrics in Table 6.1 that have fuzzy implementation (column "Fuzzy"). More about the fuzzy implementation of the metrics is available in [4].

In the remainder of this section, two experiments regarding fuzzy metrics are presented. In Sect. 6.3.1, the sensitivity of metrics to fuzzification is investigated by considering for each metric the discrepancy of similarities measured in two cases: the first is when binary segmentations are compared, and the second is when fuzzy representations of the same segmentation are compared. In Sect. 6.3.2, the impact of comparing segmentations of different types (fuzzy and binary) on the evaluation results is investigated, e.g. it is tested whether using binary ground truth to validate the fuzzy segmentation using fuzzy metrics has a negative impact on the evaluation result compared with using a binary representation of the segmentations by cutting them at a threshold of 0.5 as a prior step.

6.3.1 Metric Sensitivity Against Fuzzification

The aim of this experiment is to infer how invariant metrics are against fuzzification of images. To this end, we compare each binary volume in the silver corpus (BSGT) with its corresponding volume from the fuzzy silver corpus (FSGT) using each of the 16 metrics for which fuzzy implementations exist. This results in 16 metric values (similarities and distances) per comparison (segmentation pair), which are then averaged over all pairs to get 16 average metric values, presented in Fig. 6.2. The assumption is that metrics that measure less average discrepancy between the binary volumes and their fuzzy variants are more invariant against fuzzification.

Results in Fig. 6.2 show that metrics are differently invariant against fuzzification, that is, they have different capabilities in discovering changes due to fuzzification. Metrics that include the true negatives (TN) in their definitions (e.g. ARI, ACU and TNR) are in general less sensitive to fuzzification, in contrast to other metrics not considering the TN, such as DICE, KAP and JAC. Also, one can observe that the discrepancy metrics FPR, PBD and VOI are also invariant against fuzzification because they provide very small distances ($<< 0.02$ voxel) between binary images and their corresponding smoothed images.

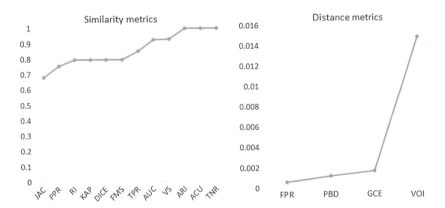

Fig. 6.2 The average similarity between binary volumes and their corresponding fuzzy variant

6.3.2 *Ranking Systems Using Binary/Fuzzy Ground Truth*

The aim of this experiment is to infer how system rankings, using metrics, change when using fuzzy instead of binary ground truth in two cases: when the segmentations being evaluated are binary (Case i and Case ii) and when they are fuzzy (Case iii and Case iv). The segmentations that were used in this experiment are BGT, FGT, BAS and FAS. Figures 6.3, 6.4 and 6.5 show the results of the experiment performed for three selected metrics, namely Dice coefficient (DICE), interclass correlation (ICC) and adjusted Rand index (ARI), respectively. The three metrics are selected to represent three different metric categories in Table 6.1 for which fuzzy implementations exist. There are seven systems (Systems A to L) to be ranked according to their performance, which is measured by average quality of the segmentations produced by these systems, i.e. the metric values resulting from comparing these segmentations with the corresponding ground truth. The averages are built separately for each of the seven organs (left kidney, right kidney, liver, left lung, right lung, left psoas major muscle and right psoas major muscle), which means the systems are ranked for each organ separately. The participating algorithms B to L produce only binary volumes, whereas Algorithm A produces only fuzzy segmentations.

The ranking is performed in three different configurations: in the first, which we denote by "binary GT", the ground truth is binary (BGT) and the segmentations are unchanged (fuzzy for Algorithm A and binary otherwise). This covers Case i and Case iii. In the second configuration, which we denote by "fuzzy GT", the ground truth is fuzzy (FGT) and the segmentations are unchanged. This covers Case ii and Case iv. In the third configuration, denoted by "threshold at 0.5", the fuzzy segmentations of Algorithm A are cut at a 0.5 threshold to get binary representations. The other binary segmentations and the ground truth are unchanged; thus, all images involved in this case are binary. In the first and second configurations, fuzzy evaluation metrics are used, whereas in the third configuration, binary evaluation metrics (threshold evaluation) are used.

In the figures, we included standard deviation columns and a standard deviation row to indicate the discrepancy (deviation) between the algorithms as well as between the three cases.

The first observation is regarding Algorithm A, which produces fuzzy segmentations. Here, Algorithm A has the best ranking when the corresponding segmentations are evaluated using a 0.5 threshold or against a fuzzy ground truth, but it has a considerable disadvantage when using the binary ground truth. Thus, it is strongly recommended to use a threshold option when the segmentations/ground truth is mixed in terms of binary and fuzzy modes. The second observation is that the sensitivity in the resulting rankings is dependent on the deviations between the average scores of the systems; the lower the deviation, the more the rankings change between the three cases. That is, if the algorithms are similar in their performance, then using a binary instead of a fuzzy ground truth, or the opposite, has a considerable impact on the system ranking. For example, the average scores of the systems have the highest deviation with kidney and liver, so the rankings of the systems are exactly the same

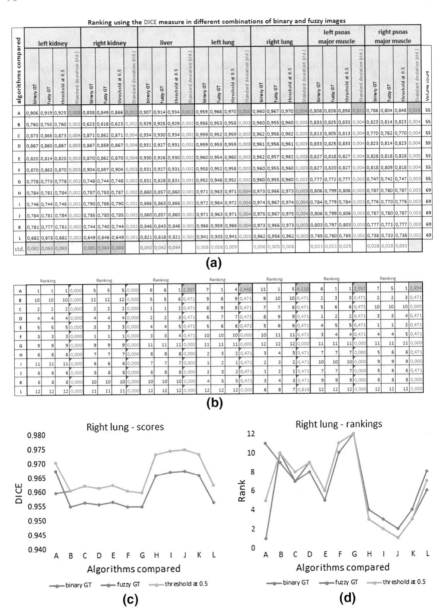

Fig. 6.3 **a** Validating segmentations using the DICE in three different combinations of binary/fuzzy segmentations. The standard deviations of the scores are to show the quality variance between the algorithms and the score variance between the combinations. **b** The resulting system ranking. **c** Score details of the right lung as a selected case. **d** The resulting system ranking for the right lung

Ranking using the interclass Correlation (ICC) measure in different combinations of binary and fuzzy images

algorithms compared	left kidney				right kidney				liver				left lung				right lung				left psoas major muscle				right psoas major muscle				Volume count
	binary GT	fuzzy GT	threshold at 0.5	Standard deviation (std.)	binary GT	fuzzy GT	threshold at 0.5	Standard deviation (std.)	binary GT	fuzzy GT	threshold at 0.5	Standard deviation (std.)	binary GT	fuzzy GT	threshold at 0.5	Standard deviation (std.)	binary GT	fuzzy GT	threshold at 0.5	Standard deviation (std.)	binary GT	fuzzy GT	threshold at 0.5	Standard deviation (std.)	binary GT	fuzzy GT	threshold at 0.5	Standard deviation (std.)	
A	0,940	0,958	0,925	0,013	0,885	0,905	0,866	0,016	0,945	0,956	0,934	0,005	0,976	0,985	0,970	0,008	0,975	0,983	0,970	0,005	0,880	0,906	0,858	0,020	0,866	0,891	0,848	0,016	55
B	0,760	0,776	0,760	0,008	0,623	0,635	0,623	0,006	0,929	0,940	0,929	0,005	0,958	0,966	0,958	0,004	0,960	0,968	0,960	0,004	0,833	0,857	0,833	0,011	0,823	0,847	0,823	0,011	55
C	0,873	0,888	0,873	0,007	0,871	0,885	0,871	0,007	0,934	0,944	0,934	0,005	0,959	0,966	0,959	0,004	0,962	0,969	0,962	0,003	0,813	0,838	0,813	0,012	0,770	0,794	0,770	0,011	55
D	0,867	0,883	0,867	0,007	0,867	0,881	0,867	0,007	0,931	0,942	0,931	0,005	0,959	0,967	0,959	0,004	0,961	0,969	0,961	0,003	0,833	0,857	0,833	0,011	0,823	0,846	0,823	0,011	55
E	0,820	0,834	0,820	0,006	0,870	0,884	0,870	0,007	0,930	0,941	0,930	0,005	0,960	0,968	0,960	0,004	0,962	0,969	0,962	0,003	0,827	0,850	0,827	0,011	0,828	0,851	0,828	0,011	55
F	0,870	0,886	0,870	0,008	0,904	0,921	0,904	0,008	0,931	0,941	0,931	0,005	0,958	0,966	0,958	0,004	0,960	0,968	0,960	0,004	0,827	0,851	0,827	0,011	0,818	0,842	0,818	0,011	55
G	0,778	0,795	0,778	0,008	0,748	0,765	0,748	0,008	0,831	0,842	0,831	0,005	0,952	0,962	0,952	0,004	0,960	0,968	0,960	0,004	0,777	0,801	0,777	0,011	0,747	0,770	0,747	0,011	55
H	0,784	0,800	0,784	0,007	0,787	0,803	0,787	0,007	0,860	0,871	0,860	0,005	0,971	0,977	0,971	0,003	0,973	0,979	0,973	0,003	0,806	0,828	0,806	0,010	0,787	0,809	0,787	0,010	69
I	0,746	0,760	0,746	0,006	0,790	0,806	0,790	0,008	0,866	0,877	0,866	0,005	0,972	0,978	0,972	0,003	0,974	0,980	0,974	0,003	0,784	0,804	0,784	0,009	0,776	0,796	0,776	0,009	69
J	0,784	0,800	0,784	0,007	0,785	0,802	0,785	0,008	0,860	0,871	0,860	0,005	0,971	0,977	0,971	0,003	0,975	0,980	0,975	0,003	0,806	0,828	0,806	0,010	0,787	0,809	0,787	0,010	69
K	0,781	0,799	0,781	0,008	0,744	0,763	0,744	0,009	0,846	0,858	0,846	0,005	0,966	0,973	0,966	0,003	0,973	0,979	0,973	0,003	0,803	0,828	0,803	0,012	0,777	0,802	0,777	0,012	69
L	0,682	0,700	0,682	0,008	0,649	0,668	0,649	0,009	0,821	0,832	0,821	0,005	0,941	0,950	0,941	0,004	0,962	0,970	0,962	0,004	0,765	0,792	0,765	0,013	0,738	0,765	0,738	0,013	69
std.	0,067	0,067	0,065		0,088	0,088	0,086		0,045	0,044	0,044		0,009	0,009	0,009		0,006	0,006	0,006		0,029	0,030	0,025		0,036	0,036	0,033		

(a)

	Ranking				Ranking				Ranking				Ranking				Ranking				Ranking				Ranking			
A	1	1	1	0,000	2	2	5	1,414	1	1	1	0,000	1	1	4	1,414	1	1	5	1,886	1	1	1	0,000	1	1	1	0,000
B	10	10	10	0,000	12	12	12	0,000	6	6	6	0,000	9	8	9	0,471	10	11	10	0,471	3	3	3	0,000	3	3	3	0,000
C	2	2	2	0,000	3	3	2	0,471	2	2	2	0,000	8	9	8	0,471	8	8	8	0,000	6	6	6	0,000	10	10	10	0,000
D	4	4	4	0,000	5	5	4	0,471	3	3	3	0,000	7	7	7	0,000	9	9	9	0,000	2	2	2	0,000	4	4	4	0,000
E	5	5	5	0,000	4	4	3	0,471	5	5	5	0,000	6	6	6	0,000	6	7	6	0,471	5	5	5	0,000	2	2	2	0,000
F	3	3	3	0,000	1	1	1	0,000	4	4	4	0,000	10	10	10	0,000	11	12	11	0,471	4	4	4	0,000	5	5	5	0,000
G	9	9	9	0,000	9	9	9	0,000	11	11	11	0,000	11	11	11	0,000	12	10	12	0,943	11	11	11	0,000	11	11	11	0,000
H	6	6	6	0,000	7	7	7	0,000	8	8	8	0,000	3	3	2	0,471	4	4	3	0,471	7	8	7	0,471	6	6	6	0,000
I	11	11	11	0,000	6	6	6	0,000	7	7	7	0,000	2	2	1	0,471	3	3	2	0,471	10	10	10	0,000	9	9	9	0,000
J	6	6	6	0,000	8	8	8	0,000	8	8	8	0,000	3	3	2	0,471	2	2	1	0,471	8	7	8	0,471	6	6	6	0,000
K	8	8	8	0,000	10	10	10	0,000	10	10	10	0,000	5	5	5	0,000	4	4	3	0,943	9	7	9	0,943	8	8	8	0,000
L	12	12	12	0,000	11	11	11	0,000	12	12	12	0,000	12	12	12	0,000	7	6	7	0,471	12	12	12	0,000	12	12	12	0,000

(b)

Right lung - scores

Interclass Correlation (ICC): 0.990, 0.985, 0.980, 0.975, 0.970, 0.965, 0.960, 0.955, 0.950, 0.945

Algorithms compared: A B C D E F G H I J K L

—●— binary GT   —●— fuzzy GT   —●— threshold at 0.5

(c)

Right lung - rankings

Rank: 12, 10, 8, 6, 4, 2, 0

Algorithms compared: A B C D E F G H I J K L

—●— binary GT   —●— fuzzy GT   —●— threshold at 0.5

(d)

Fig. 6.4 The results of the same experiment as in Fig. 6.3, but performed using the interclass correlation (ICC) as an evaluation metric

in the three cases. On the contrary, system average scores have low deviations with lungs and psoas major muscles; therefore, the rankings of the systems considerably change between the three cases. We recommend therefore to take the score deviations into account when there are mixed fuzzy and binary segmentations/ground truth.

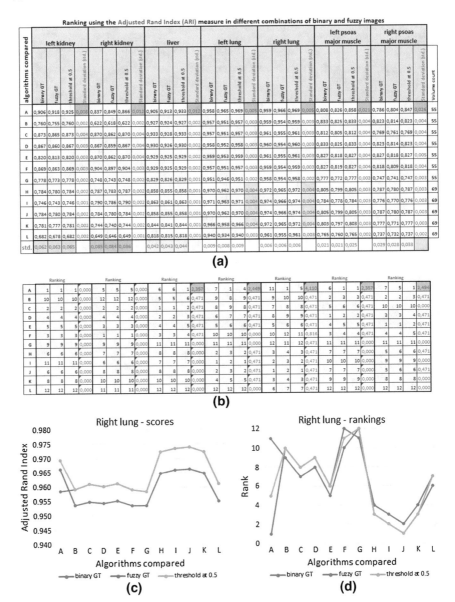

Fig. 6.5 The results of the same experiment as in Fig. 6.3, but performed using the adjusted Rand index (ARI) as an evaluation metric

6.4 Analysis of Metrics Using Manual Rankings

In this section, we provide an analysis of the metrics based on the two manual rankings of segmentations, done by two medical experts. Manual rankings provide a reference for judging metrics and evaluation methods. That is, when evaluating segmentations by comparing them with the corresponding ground truth using distance or similarity metrics, one gets scores denoting how similar or different the segmentations are from the ground truth. However, since different metrics provide different scores, which produce different rankings, the aim of this analysis is to find the metric(s) with the highest correlation with the manual rankings. Another aim of this analysis is to validate the selection of the subset of four metrics from Table 6.1 used for the evaluation of medical image segmentation in the VISCERAL Anatomy 1, 2 and 3 Benchmarks.

In Sect. 6.4.1, we describe the dataset that has been manually ranked and the ranking methodology used. We then analyse the correlation between the manual ranking and the rankings produced by metrics: in Sect. 6.4.2, the ranking is done at segmentation level, while in Sect. 6.4.3, the ranking is done at system level. Finally, we discuss the results of the manual ranking analysis in Sect. 6.4.4.

6.4.1 Dataset

To provide a manual ranking, 483 segmentations were selected by medical experts from the output of the Anatomy 2 Benchmark participant algorithms. This segmentation set has the following properties:

- The segmentations correspond to six organs/structures, namely liver, pancreas, urinary bladder, aorta, left lung and right kidney. These structures were selected by medical experts so that they cover different sizes, shapes and boundary complexities.
- The segmentations correspond to 110 different volumes each representing a medical case, where a medical case is defined as an anatomical structure in a particular ground truth volume (e.g. the liver in each ground truth is considered a different medical case).
- The segmentations were produced by seven participating algorithms. However, different volumes (medical cases) were segmented by different numbers of algorithms. This means that for some volumes, seven segmentations are available, but for other volumes, there are fewer than seven. For the ranking analysis, only those volumes were considered for which at least three segmentations are available. These are only 92 volumes.

The segmentations described above have been ranked by two different radiologists separately, resulting in two different rankings, which we call Manual Ranking 1

Table 6.2 Criteria for the subjective scoring system used for manual ranking

Score	Ranking criteria
1	Severe deviation to other organs, no connection with expected organ segmentation
2	Evident crossing of organ border, organ parts missing from segmentation
3	Irregular segmentation with respect to manual segmentation guidelines
4	Minor deviations from segmentation guidelines
5	Optimal segmentation, organ borders and adherence to segmentation guidelines

(MRK1) and Manual Ranking 2 (MRK2). The ranking was performed in a double-blind way. The ranking criteria in Table 6.2 have been considered.

In each of the manual rankings, all segmentations corresponding to the same medical case were considered as one group, within which these segmentations are ranked using the criteria in Table 6.2.

Note that according to this ranking system, different segmentations may have the same rank. For example, it is common with manual ranking that five segmentations are ranked with 1, 2, 2, 2, 3, which is not common in case of ranking based on metric values except if the metric values are discretized.

In order to test how the two manual rankers agree, the Pearson correlation coefficient between the two manual rankings was measured. The correlation between the manual rankings, RNK1 and RNK1, is 0.62. This is a moderate correlation, which means that there is a non-negligible discrepancy between the manual rankings.

6.4.2 Manual Versus Metric Rankings at Segmentation Level

We analyse the correlation between rankings of groups of segmentations produced by each of the metrics in Table 6.1 and rankings of the same segmentations based on the manual rankings (MRK1 and MRK2). This analysis is to infer which metrics have the most correlation with the manual ranking.

The rankings in this experiment are at segmentation level, which means that individual segmentations corresponding to the same medical case are ranked. To this end, the segmentations were grouped so that each group consists of a medical case and the corresponding segmentations. The segmentations in each group are then ranked using each of the metrics by comparing each of the segmentations with its corresponding ground truth. The segmentation with the lowest match is given the lowest rank, and the best match is given the highest rank. This is in order to get a ranking that is comparable with the manual ranking.

Table 6.3 shows the correlations between each of the metrics presented in Table 6.1 and each of the manual rankings, RNK1 and RNK2. The metrics are sorted according to the correlation with RNK1. Note that the highest correlation value (0.64) is a moderate correlation, and many of the metrics have weak correlation. This is

Table 6.3 Pearson correlation coefficient (CORR.) between each of the metrics presented in Table 6.1 and the manual rankings MRK1 and MRK2 at segmentation level. The metrics are sorted according to the decreasing correlation

Manual Ranking 1 (MRNK 1)			Manual Ranking 2 (MRNK 2)		
Metric		CORR.	Metric		CORR.
Average distance	AVD	0.57	Rand index	RI	0.56
Adjusted Rand index	ARI	0.54	Variation of information	VOI	0.56
Dice	DICE	0.54	Average distance	AVD	0.56
F-measure	FMS	0.54	Accuracy	ACU	0.56
Interclass correlation	ICC	0.54	Global consistency error	GCE	0.55
Cohen's kappa	KAP	0.54	Adjusted Rand index	ARI	0.52
Probabilistic distance	PBD	0.54	Dice	DICE	0.52
Rand index	RI	0.54	F-measure	FMS	0.52
Jaccard index	JAC	0.54	Interclass correlation	ICC	0.52
Accuracy	ACU	0.53	Cohen's kappa	KAP	0.52
Variation of information	VOI	0.53	Jaccard index	JAC	0.52
Global consistency error	GCE	0.53	Probabilistic distance	PBD	0.51
Mutual information	MI	0.47	Mutual information	MI	0.46
Mahalanobis distance	MHD	0.44	Mahalanobis distance	MHD	0.41
Hausdorff distance	HD	0.43	Hausdorff distance	HD	0.40
Area under ROC curve	AUC	0.39	Positive predictive value	PPR	0.38
True-positive rate (sensitivity)	TPR	0.39	Area under ROC curve	AUC	0.36
Volumetric similarity	VS	0.27	True-positive rate (sensitivity)	TPR	0.36
Positive predictive value	PPR	0.27	Volumetric similarity	VS	0.30
Fallout	FPR	0.17	Fallout	FPR	0.26
True-negative rate (specificity)	TNR	0.17	True-negative rate (specificity)	TNR	0.26

expected, since ranking at segmentation level using the metrics considers very small changes, which do not necessarily reflect an improvement, e.g. differences caused by chance. For this reason, we provide another correlation analysis at system level, in Sect. 6.4.3, that uses significance testing to decide whether one system has better performance than another.

6.4.3 Manual Versus Metric Rankings at System Level

In this experiment, the evaluation metrics in Table 6.1 are validated by considering the system (algorithm) rankings produced by these metrics. In contrast to the ranking at segmentation level in Sect. 6.4.2, here the systems are ranked based on averages of the metrics of segmentations produced by these systems. In particular, for each metric, (i) we build a system ranking by comparing metric values of the segmentations produced by the systems using significance testing, and (ii) we calculate the correlation between this ranking and a system ranking based on the manual ranks. The resulting correlation for each metric is used as a quality measure of the metric, i.e. the best metrics are those having the highest correlation with the manual ranking. In the remainder of this section, the experiment is described and discussed in detail.

Validating a particular metric using a manual ranking goes in the following steps: Separately for each organ, the average of the metric values for each system is calculated, i.e. the metric values of all segmentations corresponding to a particular organ and produced by a particular system are averaged. We denote the resulting average by the system score for the organ considered. This system score is used to build a system ranking as discussed below. Note that although each organ is considered separately, it is different from the experiment in Sect. 6.4.2 (at segmentation level) because here we are averaging the metric values of more than one medical case, all of them corresponding to the same organ, but in different volumes.

Based on these system scores, the systems are ranked using a significance test (the sign test) to ensure that the difference between the system scores is significant. To this end, the systems are sorted according to their average scores ascending. Then, the ranks are given as follows: starting with the first system S_1 having the lowest system score, it is given the rank 1. Then, for each next system S_i, if there is a significant difference to the previous system S_{i-1}, according to a sign test, then S_i is assigned the next rank; otherwise, it is assigned the same rank as S_{i-1}.

Now, we want to judge the resulting ranking using each of the manual rankings as ground truth. However, the manual rankings available are at segmentation level. Therefore, the manual ranks are averaged analogously over all segmentations produced by a particular system corresponding to the organ considered. The resulting averages of the manual ranks are used to build a ground truth system ranking using the same method as with the metric ranking (i.e. significance sign test). Now, the correlation between the two rankings (system ranking based on the metrics and system ranking based on the manual ranks) is calculated. Since each organ is considered separately, we get a correlation value per organ for each metric, which are averaged to get the overall correlation of the metric.

Table 6.4 shows, for each metric, the overall correlation (correlation averaged over all organs). The same experiment is performed separately for each of the manual rankings (MNRK 1 and MNRK 2).

6.4.4 Discussion of the Manual Ranking Analysis

The following conclusions can be inferred from the results of the analysis using the manual rankings (results presented in Tables 6.3 and 6.4).

Table 6.4 Pearson correlation coefficient between each of the metrics presented in Table 6.1 and the manual rankings MRK1 and MRK2 at system level. The metrics are sorted according to the decreasing correlation

Manual Ranking 1 (MNRK 1)			Manual Ranking 2 (MNRK 2)		
Metric		CORR.	Metric		CORR.
Volumetric similarity	VS	0.81	Mahalanobis distance	MHD	0.75
Jaccard index	JAC	0.81	Hausdorff distance	HD	0.66
Dice	DICE	0.81	Adjusted Rand index	ARI	0.65
F-measure	FMS	0.81	Dice	DICE	0.64
Interclass correlation	ICC	0.81	F-measure	FMS	0.64
Cohen's kappa	KAP	0.81	Interclass correlation	ICC	0.64
Adjusted Rand index	ARI	0.80	Cohen's kappa	KAP	0.64
Area under ROC curve	AUC	0.72	Jaccard index	JAC	0.62
True-negative rate (specificity)	TNR	0.72	Accuracy	ACU	0.56
Accuracy	ACU	0.71	Global consistency error	GCE	0.56
Global consistency error	GCE	0.71	Rand index	RI	0.56
Rand index	RI	0.71	Variation of information	VOI	0.56
Variation of information	VOI	0.71	Average distance	AVD	0.54
Positive predictive value	PPR	0.64	Positive predictive value	PPR	0.53
Mahalanobis distance	MHD	0.47	Fallout	FPR	0.48
Probabilistic distance	PBD	0.41	True-positive rate (sensitivity)	TPR	0.48
Average distance	AVD	0.39	Volumetric similarity	VS	0.47
Hausdorff distance	HD	0.38	Probabilistic distance	PBD	0.36
Fallout	FPR	0.23	Area under ROC curve	AUC	0.34
True-positive rate (sensitivity)	TPR	0.23	True-negative rate (specificity)	TNR	0.34
Mutual information	MI	0.19	Mutual information	MI	0.14

Table 6.4 shows the correlations at system level that are significantly stronger than the correlations of rankings at segmentation level (Table 6.3). Actually, this is intuitive because the errors (differences from the manual ranking) in the ranking at segmentation level are higher than in rankings at system level. This stems from the fact that ranking single segmentations using metrics is sensitive to small differences in the metrics, i.e. a segmentation with a higher similarity is ranked as better, regardless of how small the similarity difference is. This is in contrast to manual rankings, where small differences in the quality are ignored. Using significance testing in ranking at system level solves the problem, since the ranking becomes similar to the manual ranking: only systems that have significant performance difference are assigned different rankings, otherwise the same rank. The results of this experiment show the necessity of using significance tests for ranking.

The four metrics selected for evaluating segmentation in the VISCERAL project, namely the Dice coefficient (DICE), the interclass correlation (ICC), the average Hausdorff distance (AVD) and the adjusted Rand index (ARI), are in general (except for the AVG in Ranking 1) ranked at the top, which means they have strong correlation with expert ranking. These four metrics have been selected from the 20 metrics based on a correlation analysis on brain tumour segmentations from the BRATS challenge [3], using the automatic metric selection method proposed in [5].

One observation is interesting for a further analysis, namely the differences in how the metrics are placed in Table 6.4 for MNRK 1 and MNRK 2. For example, the volumetric similarity (VS) is placed at the top for MNRK 1, but at the bottom in MNRK 2. This is also the case for many other metrics. This can be explained by the weak correlation between the two rankers, namely 0.62 (Sect. 6.4.1). However, these differences should be related to the criteria considered in the manual ranking by each of the rankers, i.e. the subjective rating of the different qualities of the segmentations.

6.5   Conclusion

We provide an overview of 20 evaluation metrics for medical volume segmentation that have been implemented in the evaluation tool EvaluateSegmentation. From these metrics, we select four metrics to be used for evaluating the segmentation tasks of the VISCERAL benchmarks. We show in an analysis on synthetic fuzzy segmentations, generated using smoothing functions, that using binary ground truth to evaluate fuzzy segmentations or the opposite (fuzzy ground truth to evaluate binary segmentations) has a considerable impact on the system ranking, if the systems are similar in their performance. Therefore, it is strongly recommended to always evaluate using a threshold of 0.5 if the segmentations/ground truth is mixed in terms of fuzzy and binary modes. Furthermore, we show that different metrics are differently invariant against fuzzification, i.e. differently sensitive to the combinations of fuzzy/binary volumes. In an analysis using manual rankings provided by two radiologists, compared to the rankings produced by the 20 evaluation metrics, we show that the correlation between metric rankings and manual rankings is significantly stronger when using significance tests, since small performance differences are mostly ignored by manual rankers. We also provide an evaluation methodology and metrics for evaluating the VISCERAL Detection Benchmark.

Acknowledgements The research leading to these results has received funding from the European Union Seventh Framework Programme (FP7/2007–2013) under grant agreement 318068 (VISCERAL).

References

1. Hanbury A, Müller H, Langs G, Weber MA, Menze BH, Fernandez TS (2012) Bringing the algorithms to the data: cloud–based benchmarking for medical image analysis. In: Catarci T, Forner P, Hiemstra D, Peñas A, Santucci G (eds) CLEF 2012. LNCS, vol 7488. Springer, Heidelberg, pp 24–29. doi:10.1007/978-3-642-33247-0_3
2. Krenn M, Dorfer M, Jiménez del Toro OA, Müller H, Menze B, Weber MA, Hanbury A, Langs G (2016) Creating a large-scale silver corpus from multiple algorithmic segmentations. In: Menze B, Langs G, Montillo A, Kelm M, Müller H, Zhang S, Cai W, Metaxas D (eds) MCV 2015. LNCS, vol 9601. Springer, Cham, pp 103–115. doi:10.1007/978-3-319-42016-5_10
3. Menze B, Jakab A, Bauer S, Reyes M, Prastawa M, Leemput KV (eds) (2012) MICCAI 2012 challenge on multimodal brain tumor segmentation BRATS2012, MICCAI, Nice, France
4. Taha AA, Hanbury A (2015) Metrics for evaluating 3D medical image segmentation: analysis, selection, and tool. BMC Med Imaging 15:29
5. Taha AA, Hanbury A, Jiménez del Toro OA (2014) A formal method for selecting evaluation metrics for image segmentation. In: 2014 IEEE international conference on image processing (ICIP), Paris, France, pp 932–936

Chapter 7
VISCERAL Anatomy Benchmarks for Organ Segmentation and Landmark Localization: Tasks and Results

Orcun Goksel and Antonio Foncubierta-Rodríguez

Abstract While a growing number of benchmark studies compare the performance of algorithms for automated organ segmentation or lesion detection in images with restricted fields of view, few efforts have been made so far towards benchmarking these and related routines for the automated identification of bones, inner organs and relevant substructures visible in an image volume of the abdomen, the trunk or the whole body. The VISCERAL project has organized a series of benchmark editions designed for segmentation and landmark localization in medical images of multiple modalities, resolutions and fields of view acquired during daily clinical routine work. Participating groups are provided with data and computing resources on a cloud-based framework, where they can develop and test their algorithms, the submitted executables of which are then run and evaluated on unseen test data by the VISCERAL organizers.

7.1 Introduction

While a growing number of benchmark studies compare the performance of algorithms for automated organ segmentation or lesion detection in images with restricted fields of view, few efforts have been made so far towards benchmarking these and related routines for the automated identification of bones, inner organs and relevant substructures visible in an image volume of the abdomen, the trunk or even the whole body. The VISual Concept Extraction challenge in RAdioLogy (VISCERAL[1]) project established a cloud-based infrastructure for the evaluation of medical image analysis techniques in computed tomography (CT) and magnetic resonance (MR) imaging. The aim of VISCERAL was to create a single, large and multipurpose

---

[1] http://www.visceral.eu.

O. Goksel (✉) · A. Foncubierta-Rodríguez
Computer Vision Laboratory, Swiss Federal Institute of Technology (ETH) Zurich,
Sternwartstrasse 7, 8092 Zurich, Switzerland
e-mail: ogoksel@ethz.ch

107

medical image dataset and infrastructure, on which research groups can test their specific applications and solutions. The Anatomy Benchmark of the VISCERAL project with its two tasks, landmark localization and segmentation of bones, inner organs and other relevant structures, has a series of cycles. Anatomy1 and Anatomy2 (where the latter includes an ISBI challenge as an early teaser) Benchmarks have been completed, and the last Benchmark Anatomy3 is an ongoing open benchmark, to which any research group can still submit new methods for their evaluation to be included in the online leader board. In this chapter, the Anatomy Benchmark tasks and results are described.

7.2 Data and Data Format

This section gives a brief overview of the data used in the Anatomy Benchmarks, as well as a discussion of the choice of data format for these Benchmarks.

7.2.1 Data

The datasets used for the Benchmarks have been acquired during daily clinical routine work. Whole-body MRI and CT scans or examinations of the whole trunk are used. Furthermore, imaging of the abdomen in MRI and contrast-enhanced CT for oncological staging purposes are also included in the benchmark dataset, since there is a higher resolution for segmentation especially of smaller inner organs, such as the adrenal glands. Accordingly, these four image-anatomy combinations are available:

1. Abdomen/thorax contrast-enhanced CT (ThAb/CTce)
2. Whole-body CT (Wb/CT)
3. Whole-body MR T1 (Wb/MRT1)
4. Abdomen contrast-enhanced fat-saturated MR T1 (Ab/MRT1cefs).

We call the image data together with its manual annotations as the *Gold Corpus*; this is in contrast to *Silver Corpus* that was generated by the VISCERAL consortium by fusing the results of several automatic methods to (approximately and automatically) annotate a large set of images. The Gold Corpus is the reference annotation to train and evaluate the algorithms for segmenting and localizing anatomical structures. The Anatomy Benchmarks focus on labelling large-field-of-view 3D medical imaging data. For the Gold Corpus, manual annotations were performed and the quality was checked by trained and experienced radiologists. The Gold Corpus was built up during the cycle of Anatomy Benchmarks, as described below. The final Gold Corpus is described in detail in Chap. 5.

7.2.2   Gold Corpus: Training Set

The training Gold Corpus comprises 28 fully annotated volumes in Anatomy1 (segmentations of organs/structures and landmarks). Although the MR annotations were only manually performed in one MR sequence (T1-weighted), the T2-weighted MR volumes from the same patients were also made available to the participants in the training set. In total, 42 volumes were available to the participants during the Anatomy1 benchmark. For Anatomy2, 80 volumes were fully annotated and 120 volumes were in total distributed to the participants. The total volumes included the corresponding 40 MR T2-weighted volumes not annotated for each annotated MR T1-weighted volume. For the ISBI VISCERAL Challenge that took place during the Anatomy2 Benchmark, a subset of the Anatomy2 training set was available to participants (60 annotated volumes, 90 volumes distributed in total). Once the ISBI Challenge concluded, the test set used for this challenge was added to the Anatomy2 training set. Table 7.1 provides a summary of the volumes annotated for each of the Benchmarks from the different modalities and regions.

Since not all structures are visible in all images, the total number of annotations are not a simple multiple of images and structures; e.g. for Anatomy2-ISBI, for 6 volumes, there are only 946 annotated segmentations (instead of $60 \times 20 = 1200$). As an example, Fig. 7.1 shows a breakdown of structures and landmarks segmented for the Anatomy2-ISBI challenge. Similarly, Fig. 7.2 shows the breakdown of segmented structures for Anatomy3.

Table 7.1 Summary of the training Gold Corpus volumes annotated for each of the Benchmarks

Benchmark	Vol.	Wb/CT	ThAb/ CTce	Ab/ MRT1cefs	Wb/MRT1	Segmentations	Landmarks
Anatomy1	42	7	7	7	7	491	42 volumes
Anatomy2 ISBI	90	15	15	15	15	946	60 volumes
Anatomy2 Main	120	20	20	20	20	1295	80 volumes
Anatomy3	120	20	20	20	20	1295	N/A

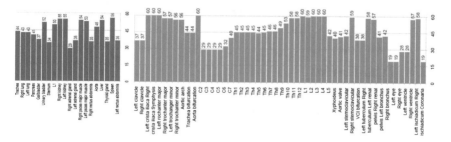

Fig. 7.1 Number of segmented structures (*left*) and annotated landmarks (*right*) for Anatomy2-ISBI

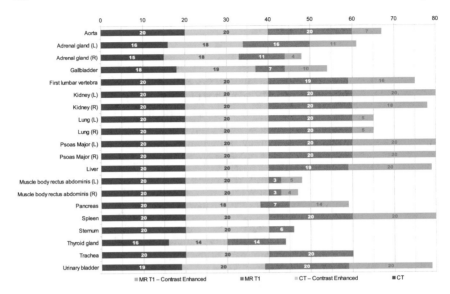

Fig. 7.2 Number of segmented structures per image modality for Anatomy3

Table 7.2 Summary of test Gold Corpus volumes annotated for each of the Benchmarks

Benchmark	Vol.	Wb/CT	ThAb/ Ctce	Ab/ MRT1ce	Wb/MRT1	Structures	Landmarks
Anatomy1	48	12	12	12	12	761	48 volumes
Anatomy2 ISBI	20	5	5	5	5	305	20 volumes
Anatomy2 Main	40	10	10	10	10	643	40 volumes
Anatomy3	40	10	10	10	10	643	N/A

7.2.3 Gold Corpus: Test Set

Overall, 48 volumes were included in the Gold Corpus test set for Anatomy1 (12 CT whole-body datasets, 12 CT contrast-enhanced Thorax/Abdomen datasets, 12 MRT1 whole body, 12 MRT1 contrast-enhanced Abdomen). For Anatomy2 and Anatomy3, 40 volumes were evaluated in the Gold Corpus test set, as summarized in Table 7.2.

7.2.4 Data Format

Clinical medical imaging is dominated by the Digital Imaging and Communications in Medicine (DICOM) file format. It is ubiquitous in hospital image management systems such as picture archiving and communication systems (PACS), and its standard has facilitated clinical integration and widespread deployment of medical informatics frameworks substantially. Notably, the DICOM standard was developed in a time of significantly different information technology environments than we typically face today. One example is the slower data transfer times that made the splitting of large amounts of data sensible, which is no more required considering current data storage and transfer capabilities.

In the VISCERAL project, we revisited the choice between image format alternatives and decided for the Neuroimaging Informatics Technology Initiative (NIfTI) format. The NIfTI format was established by the NIfTI Data Format Working Group (NIfTI-DFWG) as part of an effort to enhance and disseminate neuroimaging informatics tools. NIfTI-1 was adapted from the ANALYZE 7.5 format, and NIfTI-2 was updated to support 64 bits. Our reasons for choosing NIfTI were as follows:

1. NIfTI files are easier to handle and to exchange, since each imaging volume (or volume+time information) is stored as a single self-contained file (in contrast to DICOM format), together with the header information for dimensions and coordinate transformations that establish the link between image and physical spaces.
2. In computer science research scenarios, data are typically managed by individuals and not by central image management systems such as PACS in hospitals. Dealing with a single file (instead of hundreds of files) facilitates file management considerably, since file naming allows for a straightforward identification of files—in contrast to DICOM directory information.
3. Transferring and storing of these compact large files (which also support additional ZIP compression) is typically more efficient in newer file systems.
4. Read and write functionality for NIfTI files exists for most of the popular computing frameworks, such as MATLAB, Python and R.
5. Despite the relative ease of reading DICOM files, *writing* them for annotations is significantly complicated and prone to compatibility errors, and it is a major limitation for the development environments that can be used.

Feedback from benchmark participants also corroborated these points; data transfer was reported to be swift and easy to manage, and no complaints were raised on the choice of data format.

7.3 Tasks

There were two tasks in the Anatomy Benchmarks:

1. Segmentation of anatomical structures (lung, liver, kidney, ...) in the given image modalities, where participants could choose which organs to segment, and
2. Localization of anatomical landmarks.

Considering semi-automatic algorithms that can segment organs accurately only once they are localized (e.g. given a seed point), we also established a third challenge category, the participants of which were provided with initialization information as organ centroids (computed from the manual segmentations of the test set). We call this the *half-run segmentation* segmentation task, as opposed to the *full-run* segmentation task, where no initialization is provided. No groups have participated in the half-run segmentation task.

During the Training Phase (Fig. 7.3), the training image data together with annotations for the benchmark tasks above were made available to all participants. Participants then developed algorithms on the provided virtual machines (VM) and submitted their executables tailored for our predefined input–output convention. In the Test Phase, we took over the VM to run the participant algorithms, where the *algorithms* (not the participants) were given access to the test data (Fig. 7.4). This is fundamentally different from typical benchmark set-ups, where the participants

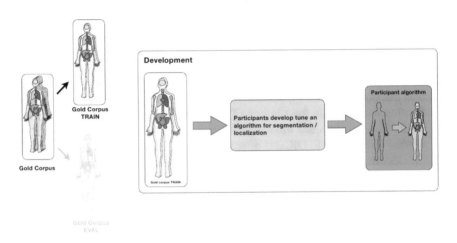

Fig. 7.3 During the development phase, annotated data are available to the participants

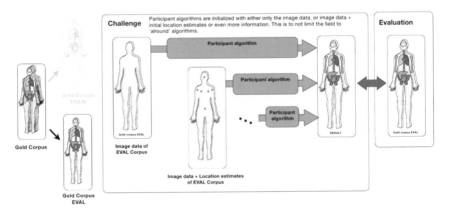

Fig. 7.4 During the evaluation phase, participant algorithms perform localization and/or segmentation tasks and are evaluated against Gold Corpus test set that is never released publicly

themselves are given the test images, where it becomes infeasible to control how much manual participant input is provided. Such release of test data also limits its repeatable use in further benchmarks or for evaluating future participants.

7.4   Results

This section presents the results of the Anatomy1, Anatomy2 (intermediate and final) and Anatomy3 Benchmarks.

7.4.1   Anatomy1

For the first Anatomy Benchmark, the following seven participants submitted algorithms, with their scores shown in Tables 7.3 and 7.4:

Dabbah et al. ($P1_{A1}$)   use a voxel-level trained solution based on classification forests for landmark detection. Datasets are first aligned and downsampled to an isotropic resolution of 4 mm per voxel. Features are the Hounsfield units at chosen random offsets from each landmark.

Gass et al. ($P2_{A1}$)   use multiatlas-based techniques for both segmentation and landmark detection, focusing on modality- and anatomy-independent techniques to be applied in a wide range of image modalities, in contrast to methods customized to a specific anatomy or modality. For segmentation, label propagation from several atlases to a target image is proposed. For landmark localization, consensus-based fusion of location estimates from several atlases identified by a customized template-matching approach is used.

Huang et al. ($P3_{A1}$)   propose an automatic and robust coarse-to-fine liver image segmentation method. The workflow can be divided into four steps: liver localization, shape model fitting, appearance profile fitting and free-form deformation.

Jiménez del Toro et al. ($P4_{A1}$)   use a multiatlas-based segmentation approach. Multiple atlases identify the location of one or more structures in the patient volume. The label volumes of the atlases are transformed using the image registrations of each atlas to the target volume. A stochastic gradient descent optimization is performed for the desired metric during the process.

Kechichian et al. ($P5_{A1}$)   present an automatic multiple organ segmentation method based on a multilabel graph cuts using prior information of organ spatial relationships and shape. The former is derived from shortest-path pairwise constraints defined on a graph model of structure adjacency relations, and the latter is represented by probabilistic organ atlases learned from a training dataset.

Spanier et al. ($P6_{A1}$)   describe a new generic method for the automatic rule-based segmentation of multiple organs from 3D CT scans. The rules determine the order

Table 7.3 Anatomy1 segmentation DICE scores of participants on Wb/CT, ThAb/CTce, Wb/MRT1 and Ab/MRT1cefs images

DICE	CT			CTce						MR	MRce
	P2_A1	P3_A1	P7_A1	P2_A1	P3_A1	P4_A1	P5_A1	P6_A1	P7_A1	P2_A1	P2_A1
Left kidney	0.805	-	0.820	0.903	-	0.921	0.747	0.631	0.820	0.730	0.782
Right kidney	0.754	-	0.802	0.877	-	0.913	0.632	0.663	0.872	0.733	0.787
Spleen	0.688	-	0.868	0.802	-	0.852	0.768	0.690	0.891	0.668	0.689
Liver	0.830	0.892	0.910	0.899	0.892	0.918	0.806	0.747	0.914	0.822	0.847
Left lung	0.952	-	0.961	0.961	-	0.955	0.853	0.848	0.965	0.533	0.650
Right lung	0.960	-	0.963	0.968	-	0.965	0.892	0.975	0.969	0.900	0.664
Urinary bladder	0.640	-	0.732	0.676	-	0.700	0.718	-	0.805	0.656	0.280
Left rectus abdominis							0.130				
Right rectus abdominis							0.171				
Lumbar vertebra 1	0.350	-	-	0.604	-	0.522	0.447	-	-	0.396	0.060
Thyroid	0.469	-	-	0.469	-	-	0.004	-	-	0.367	
Pancreas	0.438	-	-	0.465	-	-	0.155	-	-		0.356
Left psoas major	0.772	-	0.764	0.811	-	-	0.706	-	0.792	0.801	0.644
Right psoas major	0.787	-	0.771	0.787	-	-	0.633	-	0.811		
Gallbladder	0.102	-	-	0.334	-	0.566	0.281	-	-	0.023	0.035
Sternum	0.648	-	0.683	0.648	-	-	0.454	-	0.713	0.358	
Aorta	0.723	-	-	0.785	-	-	0.495	0.785	-	0.744	0.616
Trachea	0.822	-	-	0.847	-	0.836	0.696	-	-	0.736	
Left adrenal gland	0.165	-	-	0.204	-	-	0.000	-	-	0.109	0.000
Right adrenal gland	0.138	-	-	0.164	-	-	0.000	-	-	0.215	0.107

Table 7.4 Anatomy1 landmark localization scores as average Euclidean distances in ThAb/CTce and Ab/MRT1cefs images

Avg Error [mm]	CTce		MRce
	$P1_{A1}$	$P2_{A1}$	$P2_{A1}$
Aorta bifurcation	16.34	33.65	48.65
Aortic arch	9.70	16.05	-
Left clavicle	18.50	8.21	-
Right clavicle	20.65	9.36	-
Left crista iliaca	11.19	9.50	74.6
Right crista iliaca	7.80	9.35	55.92
Symphysis	7.13	9.38	52.25
Trachea bifurcation	3.90	4.51	-
Left trochanter major	7.44	4.74	66.69
Right trochanter major	7.03	4.17	77.79
Left trochanter minor	9.88	6.32	98.11
Right trochanter major	8.88	5.41	39.63

in which the organs are isolated and detected from simple to difficult. Following the isolation of the body, first respiratory structures are segmented, the trachea and the left/right lungs. Next, the organs with high blood content are segmented: the spleen, the liver and the left/right kidneys.

Wang et al. ($P7_{A1}$)   propose multiorgan segmentation using fast model-based level set method and hierarchical shape priors. Segmentation starts with stripping the body of skin and subcutaneous fat using threshold-based level set methods. After registering the image to be processed against a standard subject picked from the training datasets, a series of model-based level set segmentation operations are carried out guided by hierarchical shape priors.

7.4.2 Anatomy2: Intermediate Results at the ISBI Challenge

Participants in Anatomy2 were given the opportunity to submit intermediate results for the Anatomy Challenge co-located with the IEEE International Symposium in Biomedical Imaging (ISBI) 2014. Five participants submitted their algorithms, with their scores shown in Tables 7.5 and 7.6. Methods used by participating groups are described in these references:

Gass et al. ($P1_{a2}$)   *Segmentation and Landmark Localization Based on Multiple Atlases* [3].

Huang et al. ($P2_{a2}$)   *Automatic Liver Segmentation using Multiple Prior Knowledge Models and Free-Form Deformation* [6].

Jiménez del Toro et al. ($P3_{a2}$)   *Hierarchical Multistructure Segmentation Guided by Anatomical Correlations* [8].

Spanier et al. ($P4_{a2}$)   *Rule-based ventral cavity multiorgan automatic segmentation in CT scans* [14].

Wang et al. ($P5_{a2}$)   *Automatic multiorgan segmentation using fast model-based level set method and hierarchical shape priors* [16].

7.4.3 Anatomy2: Main Benchmark

Eight groups submitted algorithms for the final Anatomy2 Benchmark, with scores reported in Tables 7.7 and 7.8. Approaches used are described in the following references:

Gass et al. ($P1_{A2}$)   submitted a multiatlas-based segmentation and landmark localisation method in images with large field of view [2].

Jiménez del Toro et al. ($P2_{A2}$)   submitted an algorithm based on hierarchical multiatlas-based segmentation for anatomical structures [7].

Kéchichian et al. ($P3_{A2}$)   submitted a generic multilabel graph cut method, which uses location likelihood and spatial relationships between organs [12].

Li et al. ($P4_{A2}$)   submitted an automatic and robust coarse-to-fine liver image segmentation method [13].

Mai et al. ($P5_{A2}$)   submitted an approach for landmark detection in volumetric images based on the popular Histograms of Oriented Gradients Descriptor (HOG) and linear support vector machines (SVM).

Spanier et al. ($P6_{A2}$)   submitted a rule-based algorithm [14, 15].

Vincent et al. ($P7_{A2}$)   submitted a specific, automatic model-based framework for segmenting the aorta, kidneys, liver, lungs and the psoas major muscles in Wb/CT and ThAb/CTce images.

Wang et al. ($P8_{A2}$)   submitted the method described in [16].

7.4.4 Anatomy3

Five participants submitted algorithms to the Anatomy3 Benchmark before an initial kick-off deadline, with their scores reported in Table 7.9. Results from subsequent and more recent submissions can be found in the online leaderboard.[2] The approaches submitted are described in the following references:

---

[2]http://visceral.eu:8080/register/Leaderboard.xhtml.

Table 7.5 Anatomy2-ISBI challenge segmentation DICE scores for Wb/CT, ThAb/CTce, Wb/MRT1 and Ab/MRT1cefs images

DICE	CT				CTce					MR	MRce
	$P1_{a2}$	$P2_{a2}$	$P3_{a2}$	$P5_{a2}$	$P1_{a2}$	$P2_{a2}$	$P3_{a2}$	$P4_{a2}$	$P5_{a2}$	$P1_{a2}$	$P1_{a2}$
Left kidney	0.756	-	0.678	0.729	0.885	-	0.923	0.902	0.896	0.548	0.888
Right kidney	0.679	-	0.649	0.777	0.827	-	0.905	-	0.890	0.589	0.732
Spleen	0.684	-	0.677	0.887	0.803	-	0.859	0.934	0.842	0.646	0.785
Liver	0.798	0.911	0.823	0.904	0.882	0.922	0.908	-	0.887	0.817	0.861
Left lung	0.955	-	0.969	0.971	0.960	-	0.952	0.970	0.956	0.486	-
Right lung	0.965	-	0.967	0.972	0.966	-	0.963	0.979	0.942	0.909	-
Urinary bladder	0.636	-	0.616	0.806	0.657	-	0.680	-	0.738	0.577	0.334
Left rectus abdominis	-	-	-	-	-	-	-	-	-	-	-
Right rectus abdominis	-	-	-	-	-	-	-	-	-	-	-
Lumbar vertebra 1	0.333	-	0.44	-	0.548	-	0.472	-	-	0.623	0.084
Thyroid	0.439	-	-	-	0.315	-	-	-	-	0.488	-
Pancreas	0.466	-	-	-	0.442	-	-	-	-	-	0.356
Left psoas major	0.773	-	-	0.722	0.797	-	-	-	0.737	0.765	0.654
Right psoas major	0.78	-	-	0.764	-	-	-	-	0.752	-	-
Gallbladder	0.078	-	0.271	-	0.212	-	0.400	-	-	0.044	0.000
Sternum	0.63	-	-	0.712	0.612	-	-	-	0.590	0.359	-
Aorta	0.724	-	-	-	0.787	-	-	-	-	0.783	-
Trachea	0.837	-	0.855	-	0.839	-	0.830	0.856	-	0.747	-
Left adrenal gland	0.282	-	-	-	0.099	-	-	-	-	0.144	-
Right adrenal gland	0.133	-	-	-	0.019	-	-	-	-	0.268	-

Table 7.6 Anatomy2-ISBI challenge landmark localization scores as average Euclidean distances in Wb/CT, ThAb/CTce, Wb/MRT1 and Ab/MRT1cefs images

Avg Error [mm]	CT	CTce	MR	MRce
	$P1_{a2}$	$P1_{a2}$	$P1_{a2}$	$P1_{a2}$
Aorta bifurcation	19.05	36.22	252.49	61.28
Aortic arch	17.68	16.18	43.67	-
Left clavicle	9.27	16.26	13.05	-
Right clavicle	5.69	32.35	23.31	-
Left crista iliaca	7.7	13.93	23.29	88.92
Right crista iliaca	6.12	10.38	19.21	57.65
Symphysis	8.01	15.59	122.45	50.86
Trachea bifurcation	3.99	3.35	61.2	-
Left trochanter major	34.37	37.84	29.57	30.49
Right trochanter major	36.18	38.31	44.4	59.81
Left trochanter minor	5.16	11.22	18.51	28.54
Right trochanter major	4.06	12.64	62.4	34.84

Dicente Cid et al. ($P1_{A3}$)   participated with a fully automatic method for the segmentation of the lung volumes in CT [1].

He et al. ($P2_{A3}$)   submitted an automatic multiorgan segmentation based on multiboost learning and statistical shape model search [4].

Heinrich et al. ($P3_{A3}$)   submitted a discrete medical image registration framework to multiorgan segmentation in different modalities [5].

Jiménez del Toro et al. ($P4_{A3}$)   contributed a hierarchical multiatlas multistructure segmentation approach guided by anatomical correlations (AnatSeg-Gspac) [9].

Kahl et al. ($P5_{A3}$)   proposed a method for multiorgan segmentation in whole-body CT images based on a multiatlas approach [11].

7.4.5 Discussion

Participation in the various editions of the Anatomy Benchmarks allows us to answer questions regarding popularity of tasks and image modalities, potentially also relating to the (perceived) difficulty of each task/modality. Specifically, the popular modality in Anatomy1 and Anatomy2 editions was contrast-enhanced CT, followed by standard CT. Magnetic resonance imaging did not attract more than a single participant for the segmentation tasks, and only in the Anatomy2 landmark localization task, was able to attract two participants, potentially due to the relative difficulty of automatic analysis using this modality. Some algorithms were organ or modality specific, so were only submitted for that anatomy, whereas other methods were

Table 7.7 Anatomy2 Benchmark segmentation DICE scores for Wb/CT, ThAb/CTce, Wb/MRT1 and Ab/MRT1cefs images

DICE	CT					CTce							MR	MRce
	$P1_{A2}$	$P2_{A2}$	$P4_{A2}$	$P7_{A2}$	$P8_{A2}$	$P1_{A2}$	$P2_{A2}$	$P3_{A2}$	$P4_{A2}$	$P6_{A2}$	$P7_{A2}$	$P8_{A2}$	$P1_{A2}$	$P1_{A2}$
Left kidney	0.778	0.784	-	0.925	0.873	0.913	0.910	0.855	-	0.829	0.943	0.927	0.808	0.845
Right kidney	0.748	0.790	-	0.866	0.871	0.914	0.889	0.805	-	0.870	0.927	0.923	0.812	0.880
Spleen	0.671	0.703	-	-	0.914	0.781	0.721	0.812	-	0.822	-	0.867	0.684	0.659
Liver	0.831	0.866	0.831	0.934	0.934	0.908	0.882	0.925	0.937	-	0.942	0.930	0.827	0.834
Left lung	0.952	0.972	-	0.970	0.960	0.961	0.959	0.955	-	0.970	0.969	0.965	0.567	0.528
Right lung	0.960	0.974	-	0.970	0.962	0.965	0.962	0.953	-	0.968	0.974	0.866	0.903	0.725
Urinary bladder	0.666	0.698	-	-	0.713	0.683	0.674	0.774	-	-	-	-	0.709	0.205
L rectus abd	-	0.551	-	-	-	-	0.444	0.111	-	-	-	-	-	-
R rectus abd	-	0.498	-	-	-	-	0.453	0.211	-	-	-	-	-	0.077
L1	0.412	0.718	-	-	-	0.624	0.523	0.486	-	-	-	-	0.415	0.077
Thyroid	0.450	0.549	-	-	-	0.184	0.410	0.037	-	-	-	-	0.306	-
Pancreas	0.415	0.408	-	-	-	0.460	0.406	0.544	-	-	-	-	0.196	0.372
L psoas major	0.777	0.806	-	0.858	0.833	0.813	0.794	0.775	-	-	0.864	0.820	0.820	0.640
R psoas major	0.747	0.787	-	0.848	0.828	-	0.799	0.693	-	-	0.874	0.847	-	-
Gallbladder	0.191	0.276	-	-	-	0.381	0.484	-	-	-	-	-	0.000	0.043
Sternum	0.633	0.742	-	-	-	0.635	0.714	0.573	-	-	-	0.773	0.006	-
Aorta	0.741	0.748	-	0.823	0.660	0.785	0.758	0.535	-	-	0.838	-	0.750	0.525
Trachea	0.840	0.888	-	-	-	0.847	0.849	0.592	-	0.851	-	-	0.731	-
L adr gland	0.067	0.353	-	-	-	0.250	0.331	0.000	-	-	-	-	0.151	0.048
R adr gland	0.186	0.355	-	-	-	0.213	0.341	0.000	-	-	-	-	0.077	0.020

Table 7.8 Anatomy2 Benchmark landmark localization scores as average Euclidean distances in Wb/CT, ThAb/CTce, Wb/MRT1 and Ab/MRT1cefs images

Avg Error [mm]	CT		CTce		MR		MRce	
	$P1_{A2}$	$P5_{A2}$	$P1_{A2}$	$P5_{A2}$	$P1_{A2}$	$P5_{A2}$	$P1_{A2}$	$P5_{A2}$
Aorta bifurcation	35.48	79.44	-	5.83	91.83	429.13	56	17.06
Aortic arch	14.67	8.55	-	10.98	37.12	10.78	-	-
Aortic valve	54.25	7.73	-	6.48	189.02	117.64	192.35	-
Left bronchus	6.98	2.81	-	6.12	74.45	850.85	-	-
Right bronchus	16.85	3.34	-	3.87	95.08	116.19	-	-
Cervical vertebra 2	36.43	9.21	-	-	16.54	14.11	-	-
Cervical vertebra 3	17.82	12.41	-	-	127.65	11.21	-	-
Cervical vertebra 4	21.29	8.36	-	-	282.72	15.15	-	-
Cervical vertebra 5	11.33	11.04	-	-	127.35	15.32	-	-
Cervical vertebra 6	7.63	11.94	-	-	125.01	11.74	-	-
Cervical vertebra 7	9.56	15.77	-	16.7	328.86	14.63	-	-
Left clavicle	5.86	5.09	-	5.53	9.81	12.53	-	-
Right clavicle	11.09	11.27	-	8.25	17.56	19.07	-	-
Coronaria	20.33	10.34	-	8.16	-	-	-	-
Left crista iliaca	10.63	13.27	-	13.77	59.92	63.94	68.54	64.85
Right crista iliaca	10.72	11.31	-	14.84	19.28	13.44	37.35	38.16
Left eye	81.68	3.31	-	-	193.16	12.01	-	-
Right eye	75.66	2.82	-	-	192.99	1.99	-	-
Left ischiadicum	10	3.31	-	14.18	46.87	11.24	60.01	35.89
Right ischiadicum	10.08	3.89	-	13.7	40.57	9.52	70.15	35.59
Lumbar vertebra 1	33.9	24.3	-	14.62	40.67	20.28	49.57	16.38
Lumbar vertebra 2	21.34	120.4	-	6.16	55.68	9.03	43.27	11.85
Lumbar vertebra 3	28.47	23.75	-	16.4	95.44	28.07	62.16	11.75
Lumbar vertebra 4	22.14	15.48	-	16.17	89.66	23.02	56.83	20.01
Lumbar vertebra 5	23.2	11.92	-	18.2	35.43	11.94	45.07	29.68
Left renal pelvis	58.57	56.18	-	6.77	48.75	51.95	72.45	22.3
Right renal pelvis	71.83	85.01	-	20.55	53.31	50.99	45.46	43.96
Left sternoclavicular joint	11.51	3.36	-	3.34	118.18	204.31	-	-
Right sternoclavicular joint	4.89	2.52	-	3.77	143.15	122.02	-	-
Symphysis	10.73	7.23	-	4.41	191.88	13.19	48.19	53.87
Thoracic vertebra 1	14.04	14.15	-	11.1	216.69	12.81	-	-
Thoracic vertebra 2	19.86	14.62	-	9.86	36.27	60.55	-	-
Thoracic vertebra 3	12.29	11.76	-	7.07	46.46	13.84	-	-
Thoracic vertebra 4	24.66	9.51	-	9.17	81.69	14.1	-	-
Thoracic vertebra 5	21.08	39.36	-	13.21	165.64	75.8	-	-
Thoracic vertebra 6	33.18	4.82	-	15.77	137.01	9.8	178.79	-
Thoracic vertebra 7	38.44	7.04	-	17.27	145.01	55.59	156.32	-

(continued)

Table 7.8 (continued)

Avg Error [mm]	CT		CTce		MR		MRce	
Thoracic vertebra 8	55.84	12.35	-	11.85	184.15	13.35	187.26	309.45
Thoracic vertebra 9	55.86	12.44	-	19.19	139.07	20.19	168.7	163.17
Thoracic vertebra 10	66.8	12.58	-	25.32	188.43	67.44	84.32	36.62
Thoracic vertebra 11	38.77	26.55	-	22.96	140.11	15.57	85.63	18.85
Thoracic vertebra 12	32.68	20.75	-	26.6	51.38	18.93	61.47	8.04
Trachea bifurcation	4.68	2.6	-	4.94	17	9.94	-	-
Left trochanter major	4.44	4.58	-	6.27	37.06	38.84	127.11	85.97
Right trochanter major	4.77	6.19	-	3.7	64.89	97.45	68.21	71.75
Left trochanter minor	8.53	4.97	-	2.82	55.54	7.47	125.94	131.36
Right trochanter minor	6.57	4.49	-	2.67	157.91	9.13	30.6	41.91
Left tuberculum	8.45	120.91	-	12.68	17.5	53.16	-	-
Right tuberculum	11.59	7.69	-	83.16	17.6	20.11	-	-
Inferior vena cava bifurcation	16.14	10.19	-	14.14	88.35	239.12	80.31	19.99
Left ventricle	6.32	4.72	-	-	129.68	803.14	-	-
Right ventricle	7.14	5.28	-	-	116.43	1076.85	-	-
Xyphoid process	28.76	122.47	-	14.32	217.86	154.09	210.03	39.69

more general. Some participants with such generic methods seemingly pre-tested their methods on different inputs and only submitted them for the organs/modalities where these methods could actually provide a value (i.e. satisfactory results), whereas other participants simply submitted their method for all organs/modalities, whether they generalized successfully or not.

Regarding the tasks, segmentation gathered a vast majority of the submissions. Most popular organs attempted in these benchmarks were liver, lungs, spleen, kidneys and urinary bladder. Some structures were segmented by very few methods, e.g. rectus abdominis muscles.

In terms of segmentation results, the organs that obtained the highest DICE coefficient values for each modality were the lungs and the liver in CT and the kidneys and the liver in MRI. Other structures that achieved relatively accurate segmentation across different Anatomy benchmarks include trachea, aorta, urinary bladder, psoas major muscles and spleen, with DICE coefficients ranging between 0.80 and 0.95. On the other hand, thyroid, adrenal glands, rectus abdominis muscles and gall bladder have been shown to be the most difficult structures for segmentation, with DICE coefficients below 0.5.

The landmark localization tasks have shown a large variation in performance even for the same method, but accurate results with average localization errors below 3

Table 7.9 Anatomy3 Segmentation DICE coefficient on CT volumes

DICE	CT					CTce		MRce
	P1$_{A3}$	P2$_{A3}$	P4$_{A3}$	P5$_{A3}$	P1$_{A3}$	P2$_{A3}$	P4$_{A3}$	P3$_{A3}$
Left kidney	-	-	0.784	0.934	-	0.91	0.91	0.862
Right kidney	-	-	0.79	0.915	-	0.922	0.889	0.855
Spleen	-	0.874	0.703	0.87	-	0.896	0.73	0.724
Liver	-	0.923	0.866	0.921	-	0.933	0.887	0.837
Left lung	0.972	0.952	0.972	0.972	0.974	0.966	0.959	-
Right lung	0.974	0.957	0.975	0.975	0.973	0.966	0.963	-
Urinary bladder	-	-	0.698	0.763	-	-	0.679	0.494
Left rectus abdominis	-	-	0.551	0.746	-	-	0.474	-
Right rectus abdominis	-	-	0.519	0.679	-	-	0.453	-
Lumbar vertebra 1	-	-	0.718	0.775	-	-	0.523	-
Thyroid	-	-	0.549	0.424	-	-	0.410	-
Pancreas	-	-	0.408	0.383	-	-	0.423	-
Left psoas major	-	-	0.806	0.861	-	-	0.794	0.801
Right psoas major	-	-	0.787	0.847	-	-	0.799	0.772
Gallbladder	-	-	0.276	0.19	-	-	0.484	-
Sternum	-	-	0.753	0.775	-	-	0.762	-
Aorta	-	-	0.761	0.847	-	-	0.721	-
Trachea	-	-	0.92	0.931	-	-	0.855	-
Left adrenal gland	-	-	0.373	0.282	-	-	0.331	-
Right adrenal gland	-	-	0.355	0.22	-	-	0.342	-

voxels could be achieved, e.g. for the eyes and the trachea bifurcation. Modality also had a strong impact, with some structures being much easier to localize in CT (for instance, sternoclavicular joints), whereas others in MRI (e.g. aorta bifurcation and the coronaria).

Additional discussion and further information on the organization and the results of the Anatomy benchmarks can be found in [10].

7.5 Conclusion

During the VISCERAL Anatomy Benchmarks, segmentation and landmark localization methods on large medical image datasets have been evaluated. Organization of these benchmarks led to the creation of large amounts of annotated medical imaging data, which continue to be available beyond the end of the VISCERAL project (see Chap. 5). The use of a cloud-based evaluation not only represents an opportunity for larger datasets, but also impacts the number of participants. However, the series has shown that yearly cycles of evaluation can attract larger numbers of participants, when sufficient data are provided for training and testing.

Acknowledgements The research leading to these results has received funding from the European Union Seventh Framework Programme (FP7/2007-2013) under grant agreement 318068 (VISCERAL).

References

1. Dicente Cid Y, Jiménez del Toro OA, Depeursinge A, Müller H (2015) Efficient and fully automatic segmentation of the lungs in CT volumes. In: Goksel O, Jiménez del Toro OA, Foncubierta-Rodríguez A, Müller H (eds) CEUR workshop proceedings of the VISCERAL anatomy3 organ segmentation challenge at ISBI, New York, USA
2. Gass T, Szekely G, Goksel O (2014) Multi-atlas segmentation and landmark localization in images with large field of view. In: Menze B, Langs G, Montillo A, Kelm M, Müller H, Zhang S, Cai WT, Metaxas D (eds) MCV 2014. LNCS, vol 8848. Springer, Cham, pp 171–180. doi:10.1007/978-3-319-13972-2_16
3. Goksel O, Gass T, Szekely G (2014) Segmentation and landmark localization based on multiple atlases. In: Goksel O (ed) CEUR workshop proceedings of the VISCERAL challenge at ISBI. Beijing, China, pp 37–43
4. He B, Huang C, Jia F (2015) Fully automatic multi-organ segmentation based on multi-boost learning and statistical shape model search. In: Goksel O, Jiménez del Toro OA, Foncubierta-Rodríguez A, Müller H (eds) CEUR workshop proceedings of the VISCERAL anatomy3 organ segmentation challenge at ISBI, New York, USA
5. Heinrich MP, Maier O, Handels H (2015) Multi-modal multi-atlas segmentation using discrete optimisation and self-similarities. In: Goksel O, Jiménez del Toro OA, Foncubierta-Rodríguez A, Müller H (eds) CEUR workshop proceedings of the VISCERAL anatomy3 organ segmentation challenge at ISBI, New York, USA
6. Huang C, Li X, Jia F (2014) Automatic liver segmentation using multiple prior knowledge models and free-form deformation. In: Goksel O (ed) CEUR workshop proceedings of the VISCERAL challenge at ISBI. Beijing, China, pp 22–24

7. Jiménez del Toro OA, Müller H (2014) Hierarchic multi–atlas based segmentation for anatomical structures: evaluation in the VISCERAL anatomy benchmarks. In: Menze B, Langs G, Montillo A, Kelm M, Müller H, Zhang S, Cai WT, Metaxas D (eds) MCV 2014. LNCS, vol 8848. Springer, Cham, pp 189–200. doi:10.1007/978-3-319-13972-2_18

8. Jiménez del Toro OA, Müller H (2014) Hierarchical multi-structure segmentation guided by anatomical correlations. In: Goksel O (ed) CEUR workshop proceedings of the VISCERAL challenge at ISBI. Beijing, China, pp 32–36

9. Jiménez del Toro OA, Dicente Cid Y, Depeursinge A, Müller H (2015) Hierarchic anatomical structure segmentation guided by spatial correlations (anatseg-gspac): VISCERAL anatomy3. In: Goksel O, Jiménez del Toro OA, Foncubierta-Rodríguez A, Müller H (eds) CEUR workshop proceedings of the VISCERAL anatomy3 organ segmentation challenge at ISBI, New York, USA

10. Jiménez del Toro OA, Müller H, Krenn M, Gruenberg K, Taha AA, Winterstein M, Eggel I, FoncubiertaRodríguez A, Goksel O, Jakab A, Kontokotsios G, Langs G, Menze B, Fernandez TS, Schaer R, Walley A, Weber M, Cid YD, Gass T, Heinrich M, Jia F, Kahl F, Kechichian R, Mai D, Spanier AB, Vincent G, Wang C, Wyeth D, Hanbury A (2016) Cloud-based evaluation of anatomical structure segmentation and landmark detection algorithms: VISCERAL anatomy benchmarks. IEEE Trans Med Imaging 35(11):2459–2475

11. Kahl F, Alvén J, Enqvist O, Fejne F, Ulén J, Fredriksson J, Landgren M, Larsson V (2015) Good features for reliable registration in multi-atlas segmentation. In: Goksel O, Jiménez del Toro OA, Foncubierta-Rodríguez A, Müller H (eds) CEUR workshop proceedings of the VISCERAL anatomy3 organ segmentation challenge at ISBI, New York, USA

12. Kéchichian R, Valette S, Sdika M, Desvignes M (2014) Automatic 3D multiorgan segmentation via clustering and graph cut using spatial relations and hierarchically-registered atlases. In: Menze B, Langs G, Montillo A, Kelm M, Müller H, Zhang S, Cai WT, Metaxas D (eds) MCV 2014. LNCS, vol 8848. Springer, Cham, pp 201–209. doi:10.1007/978-3-319-13972-2_19

13. Li X, Huang C, Jia F, Li Z, Fang C, Fan Y (2014) Automatic liver segmentation using statistical prior models and free-form deformation. In: Menze B, Langs G, Montillo A, Kelm M, Müller H, Zhang S, Cai WT, Metaxas D (eds) MCV 2014. LNCS, vol 8848. Springer, Cham, pp 181–188. doi:10.1007/978-3-319-13972-2_17

14. Spanier AB, Joskowicz L (2014) Rule-based ventral cavity multi-organ automatic segmentation in CT scans. In: Goksel O (ed) CEUR workshop proceedings of the VISCERAL challenge at ISBI. Beijing, China, pp 16–21

15. Spanier AB, Joskowicz L (2014) Rule-based ventral cavity multi-organ automatic segmentation in CT scans. In: Menze B, Langs G, Montillo A, Kelm M, Müller H, Zhang S, Cai WT, Metaxas D (eds) MCV 2014. LNCS, vol 8848. Springer, Cham, pp 163–170. doi:10.1007/978-3-319-13972-2_15

16. Wang C, Smedby O (2014) Automatic multi-organ segmentation using fast model based level set method and hierarchical shape priors. In: Goksel O (ed) CEUR workshop proceedings of the VISCERAL challenge at ISBI. Beijing, China, pp 25–31

Chapter 8
Retrieval of Medical Cases for Diagnostic Decisions: VISCERAL Retrieval Benchmark

Oscar Jimenez-del-Toro, Henning Müller, Antonio Foncubierta-Rodriguez, Georg Langs and Allan Hanbury

Abstract Health providers currently construct their differential diagnosis for a given medical case most often based on textbook knowledge and clinical experience. Data mining of the large amount of medical records generated daily in hospitals is only very rarely done, limiting the reusability of these cases. As part of the VISCERAL project, the Retrieval benchmark was organized to evaluate available approaches for medical case-based retrieval. Participant algorithms were required to find and rank relevant medical cases from a large multimodal dataset (including semantic RadLex terms extracted from text and visual 3D data) for common query topics. The relevance assessment of the cases was done by medical experts who selected cases that are useful for a differential diagnosis for the given query case. The approaches that integrated information from both the RadLex terms and the 3D volumes (mixed techniques) obtained the best results based on five standard evaluation metrics. The benchmark set up, dataset description and result analysis are presented.

O. Jimenez-del-Toro (✉)
University of Applied Sciences Western Switzerland (HES–SO), Sierre, Switzerland
e-mail: oscar.jimenez@hevs.ch

H. Müller
University and University Hospitals of Geneva, Geneva, Switzerland
e-mail: henning.mueller@hevs.ch

A. Foncubierta-Rodriguez
Swiss Federal Institue of Technology (ETH), Zurich, Switzerland
e-mail: antonio.foncubierta@vision.ee.ethz.ch

G. Langs
Medical University of Vienna, Vienna, Austria
e-mail: georg.langs@meduniwien.ac.at

A. Hanbury
TU Wien, Vienna, Austria
e-mail: allan.hanbury@tuwien.ac.at

© The Author(s) 2017
A. Hanbury et al. (eds.), *Cloud-Based Benchmarking of Medical Image Analysis*, DOI 10.1007/978-3-319-49644-3_8

127

8.1   Introduction

The majority of diagnostic and treatment decisions taken by clinicians in their daily routine are based on acquired textbook knowledge and their experience [13]. Going through additional resources such as medical image repositories and interpatient radiology reports for medical case-based retrieval is currently inefficient and is not generally performed in clinical practice. Moreover, developing search and access technologies for information retrieval in the medical domain is still a challenging task for the information research community [3].

The VISual Concept Extraction challenge in RAdioLogy (VISCERAL) project was oriented towards improving medical image analysis tools through the evaluation on big datasets [11], and by running benchmarks in the cloud it aims to bring the algorithms and computation to the data [8]. The VISCERAL Retrieval Benchmark[1] was particularly designed to evaluate and promote improvements in the state of the art for this field. The benchmark provides a large dataset of multimodal clinical data (text and images) for the evaluation of medical retrieval and analysis approaches. In this chapter, the 2015 Retrieval Benchmark dataset, evaluated task and results from the submitted approaches are presented.

8.2   Dataset

The VISCERAL Retrieval dataset includes 2311 patient volumes obtained from computed tomography (CT) scans and T1- or T2-weighted magnetic resonance (MR) imaging. These volumes were selected from a pool of 2544 studies generated in two different clinical institutions. Only one volume per study was included in the dataset from a total of 10595 volumes in order to promote the inclusion of multiple independent clinical cases. For a subset of these scans, a list of anatomy-pathology RadLex terms (APterms) is also provided (1813 medical cases). These terms were extracted from German reports utilizing a natural language processing (NLP) framework described in [5] for automatic extraction of terms characterizing pathological findings and their anatomy in radiology reports. The German RadLex version is an older version than the English counterpart with fewer terms and a slightly different structure but many terms can be mapped from one to the other and are thus language independent. More details on the VISCERAL Retrieval datasets are given in Chap. 5.

---

[1]http://www.visceral.eu/benchmarks/retrieval-benchmark, as of 9 July 2016.

8.3 Medical Case-Based Retrieval

The general Benchmark task was to evaluate the retrieval ranking of relevant medical cases from the dataset having a query case as reference. The defined use case resembles a clinician assessing a query case in a medical practice setting, for example a CT volume, and is searching for cases that are relevant for the assessment in terms of a differential diagnosis. Ten query topics (Table 8.1) were judged by medical experts to generate the gold standard against which the algorithms were evaluated. Each topic (query case) included the following (Fig. 8.1):

- List of RadLex anatomy-pathology terms from the radiology report
- 3D patient scan (CT or MRT1/MRT2)
- Manually annotated 3D mask of the main organ affected
- Manually annotated 3D region of interest (ROI) from the radiologist's perspective

The participants then had to develop an algorithm that finds clinically relevant (related) cases given a query case (imaging and text data), but with no information about the final diagnosis of the case.

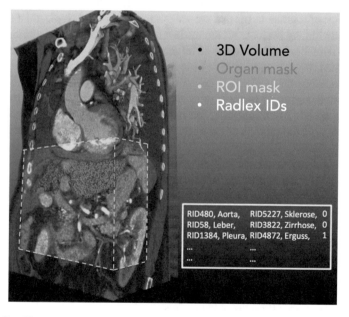

Fig. 8.1 Graphic representation of the provided data per query case. Each query topic included text information as a list of RadLex anatomy-pathology terms and a 3D volume of the patient. The manually annotated organ mask with the target diagnosis was a binary mask volume (*red*). The *yellow block* represents the region of interest (ROI) for the given case. The ROI contained either the full organ or only a region of it depending on the radiologic diagnosis

8.4   Evaluation

This section describes how the relevance judgements were obtained, as well as the metrics used for the evaluation.

8.4.1   Relevance Judgements

The submitted results by the participants were evaluated with an interface using the CrowdFlower platform.[2] This choice was made following the suggestions of [2, 4] as the interface can be used internally both without payment or with paid crowd workers. The evaluation task was divided into two parts: a task based on RadLex terms before the participant submissions and a task based on pooling after the submissions.

Relevance judgements in this benchmark needed to be performed by medical doctors, which is an expensive and time-consuming task. Therefore, a simplified preliminary task was designed in order to gather as many relevance judgements as possible before the participants submitted their runs. The task is based on the assumption that if, given a topic (diagnosis and case description), the assessors can identify a set of RadLex terms that are always relevant for this topic, then there is no need to individually evaluate all the retrieved cases that contain this term. This can produce a reduction in the number of full cases that need to be judged after the runs are submitted, when results need to be quickly computed following the benchmark. In addition, since the decision is based only on pairs of diagnosis–RadLex terms with a limited possibility to check details in the images, there is a gain also in terms of judging speed. After analysing the number of judgements received during the preliminary task, the average decision time for each pair of diagnosis–RadLex terms is 5 s.

The second task consisted in judging the relevance of the cases retrieved by the participants. A pooling strategy creates a subset of cases with the top k results of the rankings from the runs submitted by the different retrieval algorithms. The rest of the cases that are not retrieved by the participant algorithms are removed and considered as non-relevant for the corresponding run [12]. A pool with the top 100 retrieved cases by each of the submitted runs was built. The cases previously judged as non-relevant in the preliminary task were removed from the pool. In this case, each individual judgement required an average of 11–29 s depending on the topic.

The relevance criterion for the judgements was the usefulness of a case as a differential diagnosis for a given query case.

---

[2]http://www.crowdflower.com/, as of 9 July 2016.

Table 8.1 Query topics of the VISCERAL Retrieval benchmark. For each topic, the following features are shown as follows: imaging modality, diagnosis, main affected organ or region, size of region of interest (ROI) in voxels, number of RadLex terms in list and number of cases considered as relevant for diagnosis by medical experts during the relevance judgements

Topic	Modality	Diagnosis	Organ	ROI	RadTerms	Relevant
01	MRT1_Ab	Gall bladder sludge	Gall bladder	$93 \times 93 \times 52$	18	118
02	CT_undefined	Liver cirrhosis	Liver	$258 \times 351 \times 284$	12	428
03	CT_undefined	Liver cirrhosis	Liver	$326 \times 271 \times 212$	10	428
04	CT_Th	Lung bronchiectasis	Lung	$124 \times 137 \times 132$	14	161
05	CT_Th	Mediastinal lymphadenopathy	Mediastinum	$194 \times 273 \times 80$	8	248
06	CT_ThAb	Liver cyst	Liver	$250 \times 262 \times 102$	20	339
07	CT_Th	Pulmonary bullae	Lung	$108 \times 107 \times 35$	28	333
08	CT_ThAb	Kidney cyst	Kidney	$125 \times 107 \times 57$	16	336
09	CT_Th	Pericardial effusion	Heart	$273 \times 57 \times 155$	8	24
10	CT_Th	Rib fracture	Rib	$56 \times 147 \times 39$	26	47

8.4.2   Metrics

The standard NIST (US National Institute of Standards and Technology) evaluation procedures used in the Text Retrieval Conference (TREC) [15] were revised for selecting the Retrieval Benchmark evaluation metrics. The trec_eval tool[3] was used to compute several evaluation metrics from the results of the participant algorithms. Although multiple evaluation metrics were computed with trec_eval, the five main evaluation metrics considered for the Retrieval Benchmark were as follows:

- *Mean average precision (MAP)*: mean average fraction of retrieved cases that are relevant.
- *Geometric mean average precision (GM-MAP)*: mean average fraction of retrieved cases that are relevant, using the product of their values.
- *Binary preference (bpref)*: top number of relevant cases judged as non-relevant.
- *Precision after 10 cases retrieved (P10)*: fraction of retrieved cases that are relevant in the top 10 cases retrieved.

---

[3]http://trec.nist.gov/trec_eval, as of 9 July 2016.

- *Precision after 30 cases retrieved (P30)*: fraction of retrieved cases that are relevant in the top 30 cases retrieved.

8.5   Participants

There were 30 participants registered in the VISCERAL registration system. Thirteen groups had access to the data by signing the license agreement with finally four research groups submitting results for the benchmark.

Choi [1] submitted runs for text, visual and mixed (multimodal) queries. The text retrieval is based on a heuristic approach that measures case similarity with a list of conditions addressing the paired anatomy-pathology RadLex terms lists. For the image retrieval, the group used key point detection using Speeded Up Robust Features (SURF) from different sets of voxels in the images (e.g. region of interest vs. rest of the image). They then ranked the dataset images with an applied query-specific support vector machine classifier. The fusion of text and visual rankings was performed with the weighted Borda-fuse method.

Jiménez del Toro et al. [6] submitted a semi-automatic retrieval approach that generates weighting rules based on the textual and visual similarities from the query case. The main component in the final ranking is the similarity between the APterm lists of the cases, with a predefined set of rules based on clinical correlations such as same anatomy, same pathology or same imaging modalities. For the visual analysis, the images are compared using an indirect location of the region of interest from the query in a common spatial domain with the previously registered dataset. By combining 3D Riesz wavelet-based texture features with covariance descriptors, the local visual image similarity is added to the text information as an additional weight.

Spanier et al. [14] proposed a retrieval method that evaluates the similarity between cases generating an augmented RadLex graph with case-specific relations from the provided RadLex APterms lists. The sum of the link distance between term nodes from the augmented RadLex graph of each query topic is established as the similarity measure. The main organ affected is determined with the segmentation of anatomical structures in the images, and the main pathologies can be flagged by the user for the search query. This group submitted six runs using a mixed retrieval technique, differentiated by the type of imaging used in the database cases, pathologic findings, region of interest or using all these features together.

Zhang et al. [16] participated with five runs in all query types (text, visual and mixed). A co-occurrence matrix was built between the APterms and the cases for the text-only approaches. The terms were weighted by computing the term frequency–inverse document frequency (TF-IDF) or with probabilistic Latent Semantic Analysis (pLSA) to generate a probability distribution of the terms. For the visual approach, the scale-invariant feature transform (SIFT) was used to generate content descriptors for a Bag of Visual Words and was refined with relevance feedback for one of their runs. The sum combination of all text and visual retrieval results was also submitted as a mixed query method.

Table 8.2 Submitted runs of the VISCERAL Retrieval benchmark. The Type column mentions the data used in the run. A mixed type includes both text and visual data. The Input column describes how the algorithms generate a ranking of relevant cases. The Topics column shows the topics for which the runs submitted a ranking of cases

RunID	Group	Type	Input	Topics
Choi_1	SNUMedinfo	Visual	Automatic	01-10
Choi_2	SNUMedinfo	Visual	Automatic	01-10
Choi_3	SNUMedinfo	Visual	Automatic	01-10
Choi_4	SNUMedinfo	Text	Automatic	01-10
Choi_5	SNUMedinfo	Mixed	Automatic	01-10
Choi_6	SNUMedinfo	Mixed	Automatic	01-10
Choi_7	SNUMedinfo	Mixed	Automatic	01-10
Choi_8	SNUMedinfo	Mixed	Automatic	01-10
Choi_9	SNUMedinfo	Mixed	Automatic	01-10
Choi_10	SNUMedinfo	Mixed	Automatic	01-10
Jiménez_1	MedGIFT	Mixed	Semi-auto	01-10
Spanier_1	HebrewUniv	Mixed	Automatic	03-10
Spanier_2	HebrewUniv	Mixed	Automatic	03-10
Spanier_3	HebrewUniv	Mixed	Automatic	03-10
Spanier_4	HebrewUniv	Mixed	Automatic	03-10
Spanier_5	HebrewUniv	Mixed	Automatic	03-10
Spanier_6	HebrewUniv	Mixed	Automatic	03-10
Zhang_BoVW	USYD	Visual	Automatic	01-10
Zhang_fusion	USYD	Mixed	Automatic	01-10
Zhang_iter	USYD	Visual	Automatic	01-10
Zhang_plsa	USYD	Text	Automatic	01-10
Zhang_tfidf	USYD	Text	Automatic	01-10

The information that the participants provided about their techniques is summarized in Table 8.2.

8.6 Results

The results of the Retrieval Benchmark were originally presented at the *Multimodal Retrieval in the Medical Domain (MRMD) 2015* workshop, as part of the 37th European Conference on Information Retrieval (ECIR) 2015 [7]. In this chapter, a more detailed analysis of the Benchmark results is presented. Participants could submit a maximum of 10 runs and a ranked list of up to 300 cases per query topic. The 300 case threshold was defined based on experience from the previous ImageCLEF benchmarks [4], where no more than 200 results were selected as relevant in the relevance judgements. In this VISCERAL Benchmark, a few runs did have more relevant results. However, as all the participant algorithms shared this submission

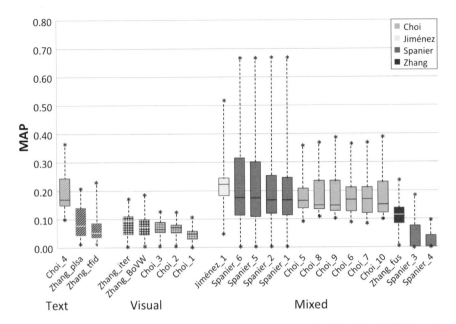

Fig. 8.2 Mean average precision (MAP) of the 22 runs in the Retrieval Benchmark. Each run is represented by a box that is extended from the first to the third quartile of the query topic MAP. The median MAP is shown as a *horizontal line* inside the *box*. The minimum and maximum MAP obtained on individual query topics are shown as *asterisks* below and above their corresponding boxes. The runs are grouped by technique (only text, only visual and mixed). The colour of the boxes is defined by the submitting group as shown in the *upper right legend*. The colour is striped in text-only runs, visual-only runs are *checkered* and mixed runs are in *solid colour*

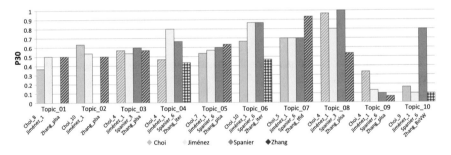

Fig. 8.3 P30 score obtained by the best run of each group, including text, visual and mixed, in the various query topics. The colour from text-only runs is *striped*, visual-only runs are *checkered* and mixed runs are in *solid colour bars*. The name of the selected runs is shown below the corresponding bar

restriction, no bias was generated towards any method. The relative performance, when algorithms are compared to other participants, was therefore the main target of the evaluation.

Topic_01
100435_MRT1_Ab

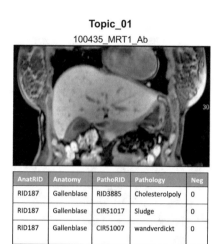

AnatRID	Anatomy	PathoRID	Pathology	Neg
RID187	Gallenblase	RID3885	Cholesterolpoly	0
RID187	Gallenblase	CIR51017	Sludge	0
RID187	Gallenblase	CIR51007	wandverdickt	0
RID205	Niere	RID3890	Zyste	0
…	…	…	…	…

Top match
101159_MRT1_Ab

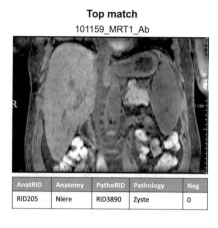

AnatRID	Anatomy	PathoRID	Pathology	Neg
RID205	Niere	RID3890	Zyste	0

Topic_04
102758_CT_Th

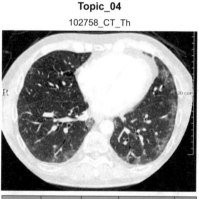

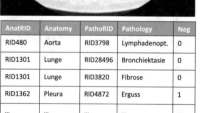

AnatRID	Anatomy	PathoRID	Pathology	Neg
RID480	Aorta	RID3798	Lymphadenopt.	0
RID1301	Lunge	RID28496	Bronchiektasie	0
RID1301	Lunge	RID3820	Fibrose	0
RID1362	Pleura	RID4872	Erguss	1
…	…	…	…	…

Top match
101223_CT_Th

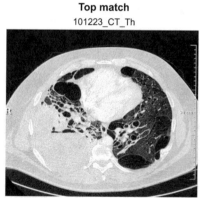

AnatRID	Anatomy	PathoRID	Pathology	Neg
RID1301	Lunge	RID28496	Bronchiektasie	0
RID1301	Lunge	RID28502	Bulla	0
RID1301	Lunge	RID3820	Fibrose	0
RID1362	Pleura	RID4872	Erguss	0
…	…	…	…	…

Fig. 8.4 Four sample query topics (*left column*) and the corresponding top match (*right column*) obtained in the ranking of relevant cases from the algorithm with the best MAP for this topic in the Retrieval Benchmark. A sample 2D slice from the patient scan includes the affected organ together with a subset or full list of the RadLex anatomy-pathology terms

Topic_09
102423_CT_Th

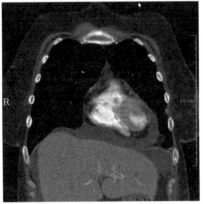

AnatRID	Anatomy	PathoRID	Pathology	Neg
RID1385	Herz	RID38588	PericardEffusio	0
RID1301	Lunge	RID39317	Infiltrat	0
RID1407	Perikard	RID4872	Erguss	0
RID1338	U.l.Lunge	RID45726	Milchglas	0

Top match
102423_CT_Th

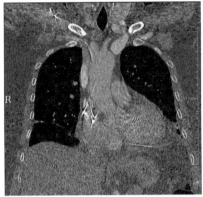

AnatRID	Anatomy	PathoRID	Pathology	Neg
RID1407	Perikard	RID4872	Erguss	0
RID1407	Perikard	RID4705	Hämatom	0
RID1362	Pleura	RID4872	Erguss	0
RID1338	U.l.Lunge	RID4526	Milchglas	0

Topic_10
100471_CT_Th

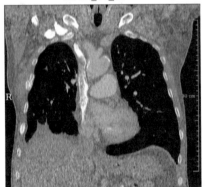

AnatRID	Anatomy	PathoRID	Pathology	Neg
RID2471	Rippe	RID4650	Fraktur	0
RID39064	Skelett	RID5045	Degeneration	0
RID1315	U.r. Lunge	RID4799	Emphysem	1
RID1362	Pleura	RID4872	Erguss	0
...	...	...	...	...

Top match
101688_CT_Th

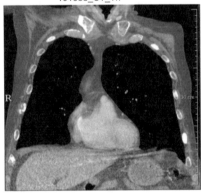

AnatRID	Anatomy	PathoRID	Pathology	Neg
RID1301	Lunge	RID4799	Emphysem	0
RID1362	Pleura	RID4872	Erguss	0
RID2471	Rippe	RID4650	Fraktur	0
RID39064	Skelett	RID38780	Läsion	0
...	...	...	...	...

Fig. 8.4 (continued)

A box plot chart with the MAP scores for all the individual runs is shown in Fig. 8.2, and a box plot chart with the P30 scores is presented in Fig. 8.3. Sample query topics and their corresponding top match from the algorithm with the best MAP score in the Benchmark for the corresponding topic are shown in Fig. 8.4. The runs are divided into three subtasks according to the techniques used for the query: text, visual and mixed. The scores from the individual runs for each of the subtasks are presented in Tables 8.3, 8.4 and 8.5, respectively. A table with the top participant scores for individual runs per metric per topic is shown in Table 8.6.

The four participating research groups submitted a total of 22 runs: 3 text, 5 visual and 14 mixed. Five evaluation metrics computed with the trec_eval tool are provided as the mean average score of all the topics (10 in total) for each run. Each run contained results for the 10 query topics, except for the approaches from Spanier et al. which submitted results only for 8 query topics (3–10). The results from this participant are also shown as the mean of 10 query topics just like the other participants. A score of 0 was given to the 2 missing query topics of this participant. The results computing the mean of only the 8 query topics in which Spanier et al. participated were presented in [7].

From the techniques that used only text, the run *Choi_4* with a heuristic ranking function based on the RadLex terms obtained the best scores. This algorithm had the highest AP score (0.2198) in the benchmark for topic 9–Pericardial effusion among all the techniques. This topic had the lowest number of cases (24) marked as relevant during the relevance judgements from the 10 query topics evaluated in the Retrieval Benchmark. The run by Choi, using only text data, was able to find the best features to characterize this diagnosis among the participants. Topic 10–Rib fracture had the lowest scores with only text techniques. The number of relevant cases for this topic was also low (47). Still, the results were better overall than techniques using only visual features (see Fig. 8.2).

Only visual techniques obtained the lowest scores in the benchmark. The most promising algorithm was *Zhang_iter* that reached 0.33 precision after the first 30 cases retrieved (P30, see Table 8.4). Topic 01–Gall bladder sludge obtained the highest scores from only visual techniques. This was the only topic using MR images, which suggest that differentiating between imaging modalities can already improve the retrieval of cases when only visual features are considered. On the contrary, a poor performance was achieved with only visual retrieval techniques when an uncommon disease, such as topic 09–Pericardial effusion, is present in a recurrent imaging modality (i.e. thorax CT). The challenge of successfully detecting and selecting purely visual biomarkers for general medical retrieval is still an unsolved problem in the literature [9].

There were two groups (Jiménez–del–Toro et al. and Spanier et al.) who submitted only mixed runs, using text and visual information in the same run. It is not straightforward to compare the influence of the visual or textual features based only on these results to the other algorithms (by Choi and Zhang et al.) who contributed also with results using only textual or only visual features. Nevertheless, it should be highlighted that these last two groups obtained overall higher scores using only textual features than their mixed runs. The overall highest MAP was obtained by

Table 8.3 Scores from the runs using only text retrieval techniques

Text

RunID	Type	MAP	GM-MAP	bpref	P10	P30
Choi_4	Text	0.1942	0.1806	0.3221	0.5700	0.4967
Zhang_plsa	Text	0.0944	0.0697	0.1830	0.4100	0.3800
Zhang_tfidf	Text	0.0810	0.0582	0.1623	0.3700	0.2767

Table 8.4 Scores from the runs using only visual retrieval techniques

Visual

RunID	Type	MAP	GM-MAP	bpref	P10	P30
Zhang_iter	Visual	0.0828	0.0541	0.1881	0.3300	0.3300
Zhang_BoVW	Visual	0.0783	0.0572	0.1900	0.0000	0.0333
Choi_3	Visual	0.0672	0.0474	0.1647	0.2700	0.3267
Choi_2	Visual	0.0661	0.0485	0.1671	0.2200	0.2633
Choi_1	Visual	0.0462	0.0188	0.1430	0.1400	0.1867

Table 8.5 Scores from the runs using mixed (text and visual) retrieval techniques

Mixed

RunID	Type	MAP	GM-MAP	bpref	P10	P30
Jiménez_1	Mixed	0.2367	0.2016	0.3664	0.5700	0.5533
Spanier_6	Mixed	0.2295	0.2137	0.3157	0.5500	0.5100
Spanier_5	Mixed	0.2265	0.2109	0.3118	0.5500	0.5100
Spanier_2	Mixed	0.2100	0.1967	0.2976	0.5100	0.4967
Spanier_1	Mixed	0.2088	0.1954	0.2952	0.5500	0.5033
Choi_5	Mixed	0.1875	0.1722	0.3082	0.5400	0.4600
Choi_8	Mixed	0.1867	0.1721	0.3099	0.5300	0.4533
Choi_9	Mixed	0.1861	0.1700	0.3143	0.4300	0.4700
Choi_6	Mixed	0.1858	0.1697	0.3102	0.4500	0.4633
Choi_7	Mixed	0.1857	0.1688	0.3097	0.3900	0.4567
Choi_10	Mixed	0.1845	0.1681	0.3110	0.3900	0.4500
hNcmJn_fusion	Mixed	0.1101	0.0766	0.2070	0.4200	0.3533
BxcvfH_3	Mixed	0.0467	0.0444	0.0604	0.2900	0.2600
BxcvfH_4	Mixed	0.0225	0.0220	0.0584	0.0000	0.0167

Table 8.6 Top scores obtained by participant runs per topic for four evaluation metrics: MAP, bpref, P_10 and P_30. When more than 1 run obtained the highest score in the Retrieval Benchmark, all the runs with the same score are shown

	MAP			bpref			P_10			P_30		
1	Zhang_fus	Mixed	0.239	Jiménez_1	Mixed	0.504	Zhang_fus / Zhang_tfid	Mixed / Text	0.600	Jiménez_1 / Zhang_plsa	Mixed / Text	0.500
2	Jiménez_1	Mixed	0.223	Jiménez_1	Mixed	0.347	Jiménez_1	Mixed	0.600	Choi_10_He	Mixed	0.633
3	Jiménez_1	Mixed	0.223	Jiménez_1	Mixed	0.347	Choi_4_He	Text	0.900	Spanier_3	Miixed	0.600
4	Jiménez_1	Mixed	0.250	Jiménez_1	Mixed	0.405	Spanier_5 Spanier_2 Spanier_1	Mixed	1.000	Jiménez_1	Mixed	0.800
5	Jiménez_1	Mixed	0.195	Jiménez_1	Mixed	0.354	Spanier_5 Spanier_2 Spanier_1	Mixed	0.800	Zhang_plsa	Text	0.633
6	Jiménez_1	Mixed	0.388	Jiménez_1	Mixed	0.491	Jiménez_1	Mixed	0.900	Spanier_5 Spanier_2 Spanier_1 Jiménez_1	Mixed	0.867
7	Choi_5_He	Mixed	0.306	Choi_5_He	Mixed	0.465	Choi_5_He / Zhang_tfid	Mixed / Text	1.000	Zhang_tfid	Text	0.933
8	Jiménez_1	Mixed	0.513	Jiménez_1	Mixed	0.631	Spanier_3 / Choi_4_He	Mixed / Text	1.000	Spanier_3	Mixed	1.000
9	Choi_4_He	Text	0.220	Choi_4_He	Text	0.325	Choi_8_He	Mixed	0.400	Choi_4_He	Text	0.333
10	Spanier_1	Mixed	0.676	Spanier_1	Mixed	0.825	Spanier_5 Spanier_2 Spanier_1	Mixed	0.700	Spanier_5 Spanier_2 Spanier_1	Mixed	0.800
All	Jiménez_1	Mixed	0.237	Jiménez_1	Mixed	0.3664	Jiménez_1	Mixed	0.570	Spanier_5	Mixed	0.638

the mixed technique of Jiménez–del–Toro et al. This method also obtained the best AP score in 6 out of the 10 query topics. However, the runs from Spanier et al., especially those using both imaging modalities and all the pathological findings in the RadLex term lists (i.e. `Spanier_6`), obtained high scores for the majority of the query topics. This was best exemplified in Topic 10–Rib fracture, where the algorithms by Spanier et al. obtained the highest MAP scores from the whole benchmark (0.6758) and a P30 of 0.8. Jiménez del Toro et al. included the visual information in a late fusion with the textual features as an additional weighting in the final ranking score. On the other hand, Spanier et al. included the visual information early in their method for the selection of the main RadLex terms in the lists from the query cases.

8.7 Conclusion

The Retrieval Benchmark was the first medical case-based retrieval benchmark using a large dataset of 3D volumes and anatomy-pathology RadLex term lists. The dataset was hosted in a cloud infrastructure with the objective to provide access to a large number of medical cases to the participants. Four research groups submitted a variety of techniques (22 in total) for the tasks. The results were compared using standard retrieval evaluation metrics. Multimodal techniques (mixed) obtained the best results when compared to the gold standard relevance judgements performed by clinical experts. The organization and result analysis from the benchmark helps address the current challenges in medical information retrieval and target the development of future benchmarks with common goals in this field.

Acknowledgements The research leading to these results has received funding from the European Union Seventh Framework Programme (FP7/2007–2013) under grant agreement 318068 (VISCERAL).

References

1. Choi S (2015) Multimodal medical case-based retrieval on the radiology image and report: SNUMedinfo at VISCERAL retrieval benchmark. In: Müller H, Jimenez del Toro OA, Hanbury A, Langs G, Foncubierta Rodríguez A (eds) Multimodal retrieval in the medical domain. LNCS, vol 9059. Springer, Cham, pp 124–128. doi:10.1007/978-3-319-24471-6_11
2. Foncubierta-Rodríguez A, Müller H (2012) Ground truth generation in medical imaging: a crowdsourcing based iterative approach. In: Workshop on crowdsourcing for multimedia. ACM Multimedia, New York, pp 9–14
3. García Seco de Herrera A (2015) Use case oriented medical visual information retrieval & system evaluation. Ph.D. thesis, University of Geneva
4. García Seco de Herrera A, Foncubierta-Rodríguez A, Markonis D, Schaer R, Müller, H (2014) Crowdsourcing for medical image classification. In: Annual congress SGMI 2014
5. Hofmanninger J, Krenn M, Holzer M, Schlegl T, Prosch H, Langs G (2016) Unsupervised identification of clinically relevant clusters in routine imaging data. In: Ourselin S, Joskowicz L, Sabuncu MR, Unal G, Wells W (eds) MICCAI 2016. LNCS, vol 9900. Springer, Cham, pp 192–200. doi:10.1007/978-3-319-46720-7_23
6. Jiménez-del-Toro OA, Cirujeda P, Cid YD, Müller H (2015) RadLex terms and local texture features for multimodal medical case retrieval. In: Müller H, Jimenez del Toro OA, Hanbury A, Langs G, Foncubierta Rodríguez A (eds) Multimodal retrieval in the medical domain. LNCS, vol 9059. Springer, Cham, pp 144–152. doi:10.1007/978-3-319-24471-6_14
7. Jiménez-del-Toro OA, Hanbury A, Langs G, Foncubierta-Rodríguez A, Müller H (2015) Overview of the VISCERAL Retrieval Benchmark 2015. In: Müller H, Jimenez del Toro OA, Hanbury A, Langs G, Foncubierta Rodríguez A (eds) Multimodal retrieval in the medical domain. LNCS, vol 9059. Springer, Cham, pp 115–123. doi:10.1007/978-3-319-24471-6_10
8. Jimenez-del-Toro O, Müller H, Krenn M, Gruenberg K, Taha AA, Winterstein M, Eggel I, Foncubierta-Rodríguez A, Goksel O, Jakab A, Kontokotsios G, Langs G, Menze B, Salas Fernandez T, Schaer R, Walleyo A, Weber MA, Dicente Cid Y, Gass T, Heinrich M, Jia F, Kahl F, Kechichian R, Mai D, Spanier AB, Vincent G, Wang C, Wyeth D, Hanbury A (2016) Cloud-based evaluation of anatomical structure segmentation and landmark detection algorithms: VISCERAL anatomy benchmarks. IEEE Trans Med Imaging 35(11):2459–2475
9. Kurtz C, Beaulieu CF, Napel S, Rubin DL (2014) A hierarchical knowledge-based approach for retrieving similar medical images described with semantic annotations. J Biomed Inform 49:227–244
10. Langlotz CP (2006) Radlex: a new method for indexing online educational materials. Radiographics 26(6):1595–1597
11. Langs G, Hanbury A, Menze B, Müller H (2013) VISCERAL: towards large data in medical imaging — challenges and directions. In: Greenspan H, Müller H, Syeda-Mahmood T (eds) MCBR-CDS 2012. LNCS, vol 7723. Springer, Heidelberg, pp 92–98. doi:10.1007/978-3-642-36678-9_9

12. Peters C, Braschler M, Clough P (2012) Multilingual information retrieval: from research to practice. Springer, New York, pp 129–169
13. Quellec G, Lamard M, Bekri L, Cazuguel G, Roux C, Cochener B (2010) Medical case retrieval from a committee of decision trees. IEEE Trans Inform Technol Biomed 14(5):1227–1235
14. Spanier AB, Joskowicz L (2015) Medical case-based retrieval of patient records using the RadLex hierarchical lexicon. In: Müller H, Jimenez del Toro OA, Hanbury A, Langs G, Foncubierta Rodríguez A (eds) Multimodal retrieval in the medical domain. LNCS, vol 9059. Springer, Cham, pp 129–138. doi:10.1007/978-3-319-24471-6_12
15. Voorhees EM, Ellis A (eds) (2015) In: Proceedings of the twenty-fourth text REtrieval conference, TREC, Gaithersburg, Maryland, USA, 17–20 Nov 2015, vol Special Publication 500–319. National Institute of Standards and Technology (NIST)
16. Zhang F, Song Y, Cai W, Depeursinge A, Müller H (2015) USYD/HES-SO in the VISCERAL retrieval benchmark. In: Müller H, Jimenez del Toro OA, Hanbury A, Langs G, Foncubierta Rodríguez A (eds) Multimodal retrieval in the medical domain. LNCS, vol 9059. Springer, Cham, pp 139–143. doi:10.1007/978-3-319-24471-6_13

Part IV
VISCERAL Anatomy Participant Reports

Chapter 9
Automatic Atlas-Free Multiorgan Segmentation of Contrast-Enhanced CT Scans

Assaf B. Spanier and Leo Joskowicz

Abstract Automatic segmentation of anatomical structures in CT scans is an essential step in the analysis of radiological patient data and is a prerequisite for large-scale content-based image retrieval (CBIR). Many existing segmentation methods are tailored to a single structure and/or require an atlas, which entails multistructure deformable registration and is time-consuming. We present a fully automatic atlas-free segmentation of multiple organs of the ventral cavity in contrast-enhanced CT scans of the whole trunk (CECT). Our method uses a pipeline approach based on the rules that determine the order in which the organs are isolated and how they are segmented. Each organ is individually segmented with a generic four-step procedure. Our method is unique in that it does not require any predefined atlas or a costly registration step and in that it uses the same generic segmentation approach for all organs. Experimental results on the segmentation of seven organs—liver, left and right kidneys, left and right lungs, trachea, and spleen—on 20 CECT scans of the VISCERAL Anatomy training dataset and 10 CECT scans of the test dataset yield an average DICE volume overlap similarity score of 90.95 and 88.50%, respectively.

Source code is available at:
http://www.cs.huji.ac.il/~caslab
https://bitbucket.org/shpanier/cbir_anatomy3

A.B. Spanier (✉) · L. Joskowicz
The Rachel and Selim Benin School of Computer Science and Engineering,
The Hebrew University of Jerusalem, Jerusalem, Israel
e-mail: assaf.spanier@mail.huji.ac.il

L. Joskowicz
e-mail: leo.josko@mail.huji.ac.il

145

9.1 Introduction

Volumetric medical images, including computed tomography (CT) and magnetic resonance imaging (MRI) are pervasive in routine clinical practice. Worldwide, the number of these images reaches into the hundreds of millions per year and is growing at a fast pace [19]. Radiologists and physicians rely upon these images for diagnosis, treatment strategy and follow-up evaluation. Currently, these medical images and the patient records associated with them are used primarily for diagnosis and follow-up of the primary condition without further analysis between and across the patients. The vast amount of information in these valuable clinical datasets represents an untapped gold mine that could support a wide variety of clinical tasks, such as the retrieval of patient cases with similar radiology images, image-based retrospective incidental findings, large-scale radiological population and epidemiological studies, and preventive medicine by early radiological detection. Indeed, the application of big data analytics to the field of medical imaging has been largely absent despite the fact that clinical imaging represents the largest single component of the medical health record.

Radiology content-based image retrieval (CBIR) is a key enabler for the utilization of previously acquired imaging data to assist radiologists in the decision-making process [11, 24, 31]. A CBIR system is an image search engine that retrieves medical records of patients with similar images from large archives. CBIR systems rely on the automatic extraction of imaging features from a non-annotated medical images database. The features include specific properties of anatomical structures, such as organ volume, shape and texture, which are automatically computed from the image and are used to compare images.

Today, most of the CBIR systems are based on global feature extraction [4]. Global features are extracted from the images with no prior knowledge regarding the content of the image, the organs and/or the pathologies and their location in the image. However, there is a discrepancy between the low-level features that are automatically extracted by the computer and the high-level concepts of human vision and image understanding: this gap is known as the semantic gap [8]. The isolation and delineation of individual structures in the images—referred to as segmentation—provides a strong shape and location prior that is expected to improve the quality of the automatic feature extraction process, thereby significantly improving the performance of CBIR systems [25, 27].

The automatic segmentation of anatomical structures in volumetric medical images is widely recognized as a difficult and time-consuming task. Anatomical structures are numerous and complex: each has unique, distinctive characteristics and shows extensive biological variability across the patients [22]. In volumetric images, many structures have similar radiological tissue properties—attenuation coefficients in CT and relaxation times in MRI—which result in very low or no contrast between adjacent structures. Volumetric images also show great variability due to a plethora of CT/MRI scanners and scanning protocols, which produce scans with very different image properties, e.g. resolution, contrast and noise.

Numerous segmentation algorithms have been developed in the past three decades. These include region growing, ray casting [16], energy active contours [3], graph cut [2], level sets [30], statistical shape model [10], rule-based methods [26] and hybrid methods [5, 9]. Additionally, a large variety of methods for segmentation of nearly all anatomical structures, organs and pathologies in CT scans have been proposed. Examples of reviews of the existing approaches for some of the main organs include Mharib et al. [18] for liver segmentation, Sluimer et al. [28] for lungs segmentation and Freiman et al. [6] for kidney segmentation.

Most of the segmentation algorithms require prior models in the form of parameter values, intensity thresholds, shape priors, atlases and a database of previous cases. Some rely on user inputs such as seeds, regions of interest and/or initial delineations to produce the segmentation. In addition, most of the segmentation algorithms are optimized for a single structure and require significant effort to transfer/adapt to new structures. Also, single structure segmentation methods usually do not take into account the contextual information of the adjacent structures which may be exploited for the identification task.

Multistructure segmentation methods have been recently proposed to exploit this contextual information [23]. They usually require an atlas of the structures of interest, which consists of parametric shape models of the structures and their relative location in the body. This approach is currently the state of the art in brain structure segmentation [1]. More recently, atlas-based methods have been developed for organ segmentation of body CT scans [29, 33]. These methods require the construction of atlases, which usually relies on the manual segmentation of the structures of interest in the CT/MRI scans and their alignment to a reference scan. To obtain a segmentation of the structures of interest in a new scan, the atlas is matched to the scan and the structure models using deformable registration techniques [21]. The drawbacks of this approach are that the atlas construction is laborious, biased to the cases that are used to construct it and thus may suffer from low specificity (the generality of such a model may hamper the segmentation of a specific target image due to the large intersubject variability in the learning cases). In addition, multiatlas-based methods require deformable registration and incur a high computational cost.

To summarize, although many segmentation algorithms have been developed, they are unlikely to be useful for radiology CBIR either due to their focus on a single organ, their need for a predefined atlas, their lack of robustness and/or their prohibitive computational cost.

In this paper, we present a robust multiorgan fully automatic atlas-free segmentation method for the organs of the ventral cavity in contrast-enhanced CT scans of the whole trunk (CECT). Our method is specifically designed for radiology CBIR. It uses a pipeline approach based on the rules that determine the order in which the organs are isolated and how they are segmented. Each organ is individually segmented with a generic four-step procedure. Our method is unique in that it does not require any predefined atlas or registration and in that it uses the same generic segmentation approach for all organs.

Fig. 9.1 The CECT field of view starts at about the corpus mandibulae (i.e. in between the skull base and the neck) and ends at the pelvis. The scan is enhanced by an iodine-containing contrast agent commonly administered to improve tissue contrast, in order to detect pathological lymph nodes or organ affection of the lymphoma

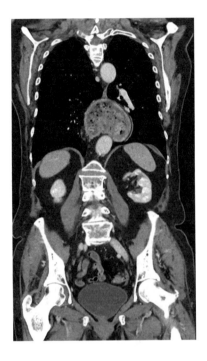

We evaluate our method using the VISCERAL [17] publicly available database and make our source code openly available for the benefit of the community.[1] Experimental results on the 20 CECT scans of the VISCERAL Benchmark training dataset and 10 CECT scans of the test dataset yield an average DICE volume overlap similarity score of 90.95 and 88.50%, respectively.

9.2 Method

We describe next a new robust, multiorgan, fully automatic, atlas-free segmentation method of the organs of the ventral cavity in CECT scans. The input is CECT scans of the whole trunk (Fig. 9.1), with the patient properly positioned on their back. The field of view starts between the skull base and the neck and ends at the pelvis, and with none of the seven organs to be segmented missing. The output of our method is a segmentation of the seven organs of the ventral cavity: the trachea, both lungs, both kidneys, the spleen and the liver. Our method consists of two processes: the first is a scan-specific characterization process that determines the grey values of the high blood content organs (i.e. kidneys, spleen, and liver), and a localization of six cross sections of interest in the scan. The second is a generic four-step pipeline

---

[1]http://www.cs.huji.ac.il/~caslab.

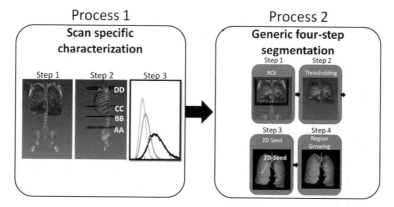

Fig. 9.2 Our method consists of two processes: (1) a scan-specific characterization process that locates six cross sections of interest in the scan along with the grey-level values of the high blood content organs (Process 1) and (2) a four-step pipeline segmentation process for segmenting each organ (Process 2)

segmentation process followed by a fine-tuning post-processing step. The method is illustrated in Fig. 9.2 and summarized in Table 9.1.

Next, we describe the two processes, followed by details of the implementation for seven ventral cavity organs: the trachea, the left and right lungs, the left and right kidneys, the spleen and the liver.

9.2.1   Process 1: Scan-Specific Characterization

The goal of the scan-specific characterization process is to locate six cross sections of interest in the CECT scan along with the grey-level values of the high blood content organs. There are three steps in this process: (1) isolation of the bone skeleton and the breathing system (lungs and trachea), (2) localization of six cross sections of interest inside the body and (3) identification of the grey-level values of the high blood content organs (i.e. kidneys, spleen and liver). Below is a detailed description of each step.

1. **Bone Skeleton and Breathing System Isolation**: We start by isolating the patient's body from the background (air and scan gantry) based on the location and intensity values. We then identify the bone skeleton and the breathing system (lungs and trachea). Next, we isolate the largest connected components that contain grey levels above 250 HU for the skeleton and the largest connected components that contain grey levels between -1000 and -500 HU for the breathing system.
2. **Cross-Sectional Localization**: We define six cross sections of interest, which will be used to define the ROI of the various organs, they are marked by labels

Table 9.1 Summary of the detailed implementation of the four-step segmentation for each organ. The rows in the table represent the steps of the segmentation algorithm, the seven columns list the parameters for each organ at each step. Abbreviations used in the table: AA—the narrowest slice of bones in the beginning of the lumbar region, BB—the inferior slice of the breathing system, CC—the widest slice of the breathing system, DD—the superior slice of the breathing system (the narrowest slice of the breathing system) and FF - the plane that bisects the spinal column at 45° (Fig. 9.3). μ_{BV} and σ_{BV} stand for the average and the standard deviation of the lungs' blood vessels' grey-level values. μ_{kmean} stands for the average of the two cluster centres produced by the k-means clustering algorithm—with $k = 2$—to cluster all voxels confined by slices AA, CC and to the left of EE and that have grey-level values between zero and $\mu_{BV} + 3\sigma_{BV}$

Steps			Trachea	Lungs	Left kidney	Spleen	Right kidney	Liver
ROI	Axial	Upper	DD	DD	CC	CC	CC	CC
		Lower	BB	BB	AA	AA	AA	AA
	Sagittal coronal		ALL	ALL	left side of FF	left side of FF	right side of FF	right side of FF
Threshold	Upper value		$-500HU$	$-500HU$	$\mu_{BV} + 3\sigma_{BV}$	μ_{kmean}	$\mu_{BV} + 3\sigma_{BV}$	μ_{kmean}
	Lower value		$-1000HU$	$-1000HU$	μ_{kmean}	$\mu_{BV} - 0.5\sigma_{BV}$	μ_{kmean}	$\mu_{BV} - 0.5\sigma_{BV}$
2D seed identification			DD	CC	Widest in the left kidney	The first slice above the left kidney	Widest in the ROI	The first slice above the left kidney
Slice region growing			Upwards to the top of the ROI and downwards to the first bifurcation.	Spectral clustering to isolate each lung	Upwards and downwards in the ROI. Between each pair of slices, the regiongrowing continues only into the largest connected component			
Post-processing, control mechanism			Post-processing includes a number of morphological operators; segmentations below 30% of average organ volume are excluded					

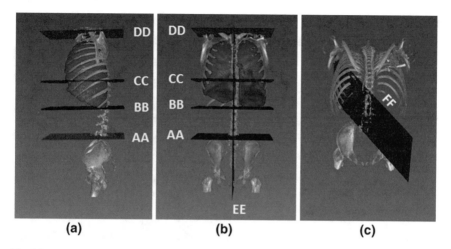

Fig. 9.3 Localization of six cross sections: *AA*—the narrowest slice of bones in the beginning of the lumbar region; *BB*—the inferior slice of the breathing system; *CC*—the widest slice of the breathing system; and *DD*—the superior slice of the breathing system (which is also the narrowest slice of the breathing system). *EE*—the sagittal symmetrical plane; *FF*—a plane bisecting the spinal column at 45°

AA through *FF* in Fig. 9.3. Four of the cross sections are axial, one is sagittal and one is diagonal. The cross sections are: (1) the narrowest slice of bones in the beginning of the lumbar region (marked by *AA*), hereinafter the narrowest slice and widest slice are defined by measuring the perimeter of the 2D convex hull in the axial slice; (2) the inferior slice of the breathing system (marked by *BB*); (3) the widest slice of the breathing system (marked by *CC*); (4) the superior slice of the breathing system, which is also the narrowest slice of the breathing system (marked by *DD*); (5) the sagittal plane through the middle of the spinal column (marked by *EE*); and (6) the plane that passes through the centre of the spinal column at 45° (marked by *FF*). Slice *AA* is found by starting at slice *BB* and moving inferiorly slice by slice along the axial planes, when the bone perimeter increases by over 200%, that slice is defined as *AA*. To define planes *EE* and *FF*, we construct a bounding box around the bone cross section at slice *BB*; *EE* is the sagittal symmetrical plane bisecting it; and *FF* is the plane bisecting it at 45°.

3. **Grey-Level-Value Identification**: We first identify the grey level of the lungs' blood vessels by isolating all voxels with values that are greater than zero inside the lungs (Fig. 9.4). We denote the average and the standard deviation of these blood vessels' grey-level values as μ_{BV} and σ_{BV}, respectively. Next, we apply the k-means clustering algorithm with $k = 2$ on all voxels confined by slices *AA*, *CC* and to the left of *EE* and that have grey-level values between zero and $\mu_{BV} + 3\sigma_{BV}$. We denote the average of those two cluster centres as μ_{kmean}. These values will be used to define the thresholds that differentiate between the kidneys, the spleen and the liver.

Fig. 9.4 Illustration of grey-level values estimation: Inside the breathing system (*blue*), all voxels that contain grey-level values greater than zero (*red*) are the lungs' blood supply. The grey-level values of other organs in the scan are estimated by computing the average and standard deviation of those voxels

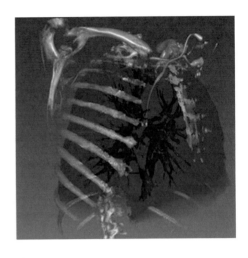

9.2.2 Process 2: Generic Four-Step Segmentation

In the generic four-step segmentation process, organs are isolated and segmented, from the simplest one to the most difficult one. Using the cross sections and the grey-level values identified by the first process, the four-step framework is applied to the organs in the following order. First, the breathing system organs (i.e. the trachea and the lungs) are segmented. Next, the high blood content organs (i.e. kidneys, spleen, and liver) are segmented, first those on the left, which are better separated, then those on the right. For each organ, the process starts with a coarse segmentation that is refined along the further steps until the final segmentation is obtained. The organ segmentation order prevents the ambiguous assignment of the same image region to multiple organs, as previously segmented image regions are excluded from the later segmentation process. We describe next the four successive steps. In addition, Table 9.1 summarizes the details and parameters for this process.

1. ROI Identification—The region of interest (ROI) is extracted and constitutes a coarse initial segmentation. This step is organ-dependent and is based on the location of the organ in the ventral cavity in the current scan.
2. Thresholding—After ROI identification, we threshold the CECT scan to fine-tune the coarse segmentation of the organ based on its unique grey-level characteristics. Note that the thresholding value derived in Process 1 is organ specific and scan specific.
3. 2D Seed Identification—A representative 2D axial slice of the organ in the CECT scan is identified. This slice serves as the set of seeds for the region-growing step.
4. Slice Region Growing—Organ segmentation by 3D region growing starting from the 2D seed (2D axial slice) to obtain the final segmentation of the organ.

Figure 9.5 illustrates each of the four steps for the segmentation of the lungs.

Fig. 9.5 Illustration of the four steps of Process 2 on the lungs: (1) The breathing system (lungs and trachea) ROI, (2) thresholding it with a scan-specific and structure-specific value, (3) 2D axial slice that serves as the set of seeds for region growing, (4) 3D region growing starting from the 2D seed upwards and downwards inside the ROI

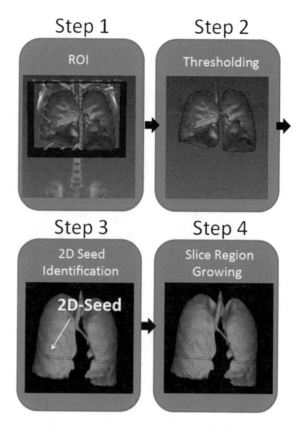

9.2.3   Process 2: Implementation details

Below are the details of the implementation of the four-step segmentation process for seven ventral cavity organs: the trachea, the left and right lungs, the left and right kidneys, the spleen and the liver.

Step 1: ROI Identification

The ROI of each organ is obtained as follows:

Lungs and Trachea: The lungs and trachea are located within the region confined by slices *BB* and *DD*, as illustrated in Fig. 9.5, Step 1.

Left Kidney and Spleen: The left kidney and spleen are located within the region defined by slices *AA*, *CC* and the area to the left of *FF*, as illustrated in Fig. 9.6.

Right Kidney and Liver: The right kidney and the liver are located within the region defined by slices *AA*, *CC* and the area to the right of *FF* as illustrated in Figs. 9.6 and 9.7.

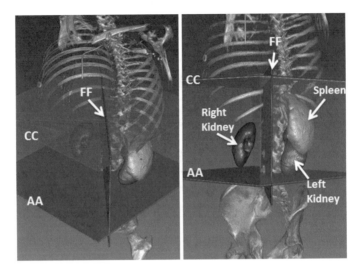

Fig. 9.6 Two views of the kidneys' and spleen's ROI. The ROI is defined by slices *AA*, *CC* and the area to the *left* of *FF* for the *left kidney* and spleen and the area to the *right* of *FF* for the *right kidney*

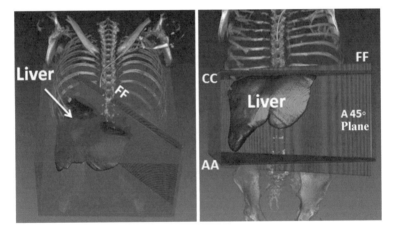

Fig. 9.7 Two views of the same liver ROI. Slices *AA*, *CC* and the area to the *right* of *FF* define the ROI

Step 2: Thresholding

We threshold the CECT scan to refine the coarse segmentation obtained from the ROI.

Lungs and Trachea: Inside the ROI, a threshold is applied to include all voxels in the range [−1000HU, −500HU], and then, the largest connected component is selected (Fig. 9.5, Step 2).

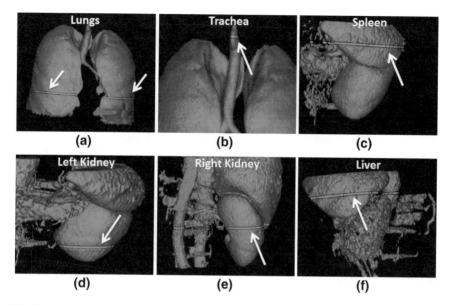

Fig. 9.8 Illustration of the location of the organs' 2D seed (*green plane*): Inside the ROI, the axial slice with the widest perimeter is selected for (a) the lungs, (d) *left kidney* and (e) the *right kidney*. The axial slice with the narrowest perimeter is selected for the trachea (b). The first slice above the *left kidney* is selected for the spleen (c) and the liver (f)

Kidney, Liver and Spleen: For the kidneys, we threshold inside the ROI by including only the voxels in the range $[\mu_{kmean}, \mu_{BV} + 3\sigma_{BV}]$. For the liver and spleen, we only include the voxels in the range $[\mu_{BV} - 0.5\sigma_{BV}, \mu_{kmean}]$. We use μ_{kmean} as the threshold to separate the kidneys, which are significantly richer in blood vessels, from the spleen and liver.

Step 3: 2D Seed Identification

The 2D axial slice selection is organ specific and is performed as follows:

Lungs and Trachea: Inside the lungs and trachea ROIs (Fig. 9.5, Step 1), the axial slice with the narrowest perimeter (*DD*) is selected as the 2D seed for the trachea. The axial slice with the widest perimeter (*CC*) is selected as the 2D seed for the lungs. Note that the widest axial slice of the lungs contains two connected components, for the left and right lungs (Fig. 9.8a, b).

Kidneys: Inside the kidneys' ROI, the axial slice with the widest perimeter is selected as the 2D seed for the kidneys (Fig. 9.8d, e).

Liver and Spleen: The first slice above the left kidney is selected as the 2D seed for the liver and spleen (Fig. 9.8c, f).

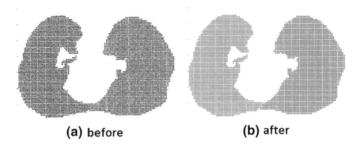

(a) before   **(b) after**

Fig. 9.9 Axial slice showing the results of the spectral cluster algorithm to isolate each lung

Step 4: Slice Region Growing

For each organ, we perform the region growing from the axial 2D seed. The seed is extended slice by slice along the axial planes, within the coarse segmentation obtained in Step 3, to include the entire organ. The unique segmentation characteristics for each organ are as follows:

Lungs: Inevitably, in the lungs, some axial slices might appear as a single connected component. To avoid this and to isolate each lung on those slices, we use the spectral clustering algorithm [20] with two clusters. Figure 9.9 illustrates the result of using the spectral clustering algorithm.

Note that the widest axial slice of the lungs, used as the 2D seeds at Step 3, occurs around the heart, which pushes the lungs out of its way, thus acting as a natural separator, so the lungs do not appear as a single connected component.

Trachea: The region growing is performed upwards to the top of the ROI and downwards to the first bifurcation.

Kidneys, Liver, Spleen: The region growing is performed upwards and downwards from the seed slice within the ROI. Between each pair of slices, the region growing continues only into the largest connected component that intersects with the current slice. All smaller intersected components are removed, as ventral cavity organs are relatively smooth, so two adjacent voxels of the same organ cannot exceed some level of variability (Fig. 9.10). This process is repeated throughout the slices inside the ROI.

9.2.4 Post-processing at the End of Process 2

A final post-processing fine-tuning sequence is performed on the kidneys, liver and spleen in order to finalize their segmentation. This post-processing sequence is different for each organ.

Kidneys: First, holes in the image are filled. Next, all connected components that have fewer than 50 pixels are removed. Then, the largest 3D connected component

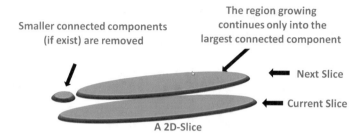

Fig. 9.10 Schematic illustration of the liver, spleen and kidneys region growing between two adjacent slices. The current slice contains a single component. The next slice contains two components. The region growing proceeds into the largest component (*blue*) that intersects with the current slice, where the smaller intersected components are removed (*red*)

is selected. And finally, a closing operation with a disc-shaped structuring element with a radius of 3 pixels is performed.

Liver: First, all connected components that have fewer than 50 pixels are removed. Next, the largest 3D-connected component is selected. And finally, holes in the image are filled.

Spleen: A closing operation with a disc-shaped structuring element with a radius of 4 pixels is performed.

Note that the morphological operators are 2D and are applied to the axial slices.

To further increase the overall accuracy and the robustness of our method, we use a simple control mechanism to detect major failures in the segmentation process. When the volume of a segmented organ is less than 30% of the mean volume for that organ from the 20 ground truths of the training set, we classified the segmentation as a failure. We exclude failure cases for two reasons. First, we follow the VISCERAL Benchmark guidelines for the results. The guidelines exclude empty files from the evaluation, so we added a quality-assurance step with a rigorous threshold to filter out these cases. Second, note that the segmentation algorithm is the first step of a content-based image retrieval (CBIR) system, the goal is to retrieve the 10–30 most relevant scans. Those failure cases are marked with N/A in Table 9.2.

9.3   The VISCERAL Benchmark

The VISCERAL Anatomy2 Benchmark dataset [17] consists of four modalities: CT and MR scans of the whole body (wb), CECT scans of the whole trunk and T1 contrast-enhanced MR scans of the abdomen. Each modality has 30 clinical scans (a training dataset of 20 scans was made available to participants before the benchmark, and a test dataset of 10 scans used only by the organizers). All scans were acquired between 2004 and 2008. Our method was submitted for the CECT whole trunk modality.

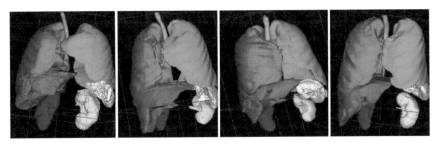

Fig. 9.11 Multiorgan segmentation results of four representative CECT scans of the VISCERAL Challenge

The CECT whole trunk scans were acquired from adult patients with malignant lymphoma. Their field of view starts between the skull base and the neck and ends at the pelvis. In-plane resolution is $0.604 - 0.793$ mm; the in-between plane resolution is 3 mm. A VISCERAL team radiologist manually produced ground truth segmentation for each scan.

The VISCERAL training and test datasets were uploaded to the Azure cloud framework. The training dataset was made available to all registered benchmark participants. In this unique cloud-based evaluation benchmark [14], the participants were required to submit their source code and the testing was conducted by the organizers. The participants received a virtual cloud computing 8-core CPU instance with 16-GB RAM. Both the executable and the required libraries were installed by the participants in the virtual machines. The test dataset was not accessible to the participants. The organizers ran the virtual machines with the participants' segmentation software on the test data. The goal of this framework is to generate an objective and unbiased evaluation of the different algorithms with the same test dataset and the same computing capabilities for all the participants.

9.4 Results and Discussion

Table 9.2 shows the results for the training dataset; Table 9.3 summarizes the results for the test dataset. The high values of DICE similarity coefficients demonstrate the reliability of our method. In the recent VISCERAL Challenge, for air-containing organs, our method was ranked as one of the top [13]. Figure 9.11 shows four representative examples of the multiorgan segmentation results.

Note that the only organ for which our segmentation averages below 90% accuracy is the liver. This stems from the fact that the liver is the most complex organ in the body, with very high variance among the individuals, and varying grey levels according to the phase in which the scan was obtained.

Our approach throughout the paper is based on the anatomical analysis. The aim of the ROIs is to identify the location of the organs defined by medical-anatomical knowledge. The thresholds for separating the kidneys from the spleen/liver are based

Table 9.2 DICE similarity score per organ for the training dataset (20 CECT scans)

Subject id	Trachea	Left lung	Right lung	Right kidney	Left kidney	Liver	Spleen
10000100	0.96	0.97	0.97	0.88	0.82	0.91	0.94
10000104	0.83	0.98	0.97	0.90	0.92	N/A	0.78
10000105	N/A	0.93	0.92	0.86	0.90	0.94	0.94
10000106	0.89	0.98	0.97	0.92	0.94	0.90	0.89
10000108	0.89	0.98	0.98	0.89	0.93	0.92	0.81
10000109	0.94	0.96	0.95	0.90	0.91	0.87	0.92
10000110	0.84	0.98	0.98	0.95	0.95	0.85	0.92
10000111	0.95	0.96	0.97	0.92	0.91	N/A	0.94
10000112	0.91	0.97	0.94	N/A	0.92	0.74	0.83
10000113	0.91	0.97	0.98	0.95	0.95	0.91	0.96
10000127	0.82	0.97	0.97	N/A	N/A	0.73	N/A
10000128	0.85	0.96	0.98	0.89	0.91	0.87	0.93
10000129	0.84	0.98	0.98	N/A	N/A	0.93	N/A
10000130	0.85	0.96	0.96	0.91	0.91	0.86	0.95
10000131	0.96	0.96	0.95	0.93	0.94	0.86	0.91
10000132	0.96	0.77	0.95	0.91	0.92	0.92	0.94
10000133	0.87	0.97	0.95	0.92	0.92	0.90	0.78
10000134	0.92	0.99	0.98	0.90	0.92	0.85	0.92
10000135	0.94	0.98	0.95	0.89	0.91	0.92	0.85
10000136	N/A	0.98	0.97	0.93	0.91	0.84	0.95
Average	**.90**	**0.96**	**0.96**	**0.91**	**0.92**	**0.87**	**0.90**

on the fact that the kidneys are significantly richer in blood vessels. The fact that the widest axial slice of the lungs occurs around the heart, which acts as a natural separator, ascertains the lungs do not appear as a single connected component at that point.

An advantage of the cloud-based evaluation framework is that it required us to develop robust and portable software, which we published as open source that can be integrated in different platforms such as the clinical environment.

If one of the organ segmentations failed during the pipeline process, all following organs will fail too. This is because of the dependency between segmentation steps. Such a scenario occurred for subjects 10000127 and 10000129 (Table 9.2), for the segmentation of the left kidney failed and as a result segmentation of all succeeding organs—spleen and the right kidney—failed. This could also happen in cases of nephrectomy (kidney removal).

Table 9.3 Results: Average DICE similarity score per organ for the test dataset (10 CECT scans)

Test dataset	Trachea	Left lung	Right lung	Right kidney	Left kidney	Spleen
	85.1	97.0	96.8	87.0	82.9	82.2

Fig. 9.12 The enlarged
spleen of subject 1000112:
In some rare cases, organs
might extend outside the
ROI; this happens in cases of
enlarged organs

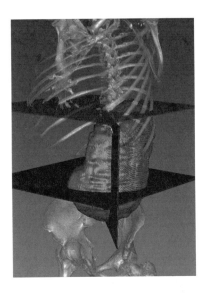

Note that segmentations 10000127 and 10000129 were tagged as failure by our control mechanism which excludes any segmentation result if it is below 30% of the average volume calculated for the organ. Working in the field of big data, we consider it much more preferable to retrieve fewer cases, but be more assured they are highly relevant cases, than to risk retrieving less relevant cases, because they were mis-segmented.

Another limitation can come from the construction of the ROI. There are some rare cases where the organs extend outside the ROI; this happens in cases of enlarged organs that vary from the standard shape. Such an example is shown in Fig. 9.12.

9.5 VISCERAL Benchmark Perspective

Five other groups participated in the VISCERAL Anatomy2 Benchmark for the CECT modality. Below is a short description of their methods, followed by a short discussion.

Kechichian et al. [15] propose a generic method based on a multilabel graph cut optimization approach that uses location likelihood of organs and prior information of spatial relationships between them. Organ atlases are mapped and used. To derive organ intensity likelihoods, prior and likelihood models are then introduced in a joint centroidal Voronoi image clustering and graph cut multiobject segmentation framework. Wang et al. [32] segmented 10 anatomical structures in CT contrast-enhanced and non-enhanced scans. Their multiorgan segmentation pipeline follows a top-down approach based on the level set segmentation of the ventral cavity. After dividing the cavity into the thoracic and abdominal cavities, the major structures are segmented based on statistical shape and their location information is used to segment the lower-level structures. Jimenez del Toro et al. [12] segment structures in CT contrast-enhanced and non-enhanced scans with a hierarchical multiatlas approach. Based on the spatial anatomical correlations between the organs, the bigger and higher-contrast organs are segmented first. These initial volume transformations form the basis for identifying the smaller structures with less defined boundaries. Goksel et al. [7] describe segmentation methods for both CT and MR anatomical structures. They use a multiatlas-based technique that uses Markov random fields to guide the registrations. A multiatlas template-based approach fuses the different deformable registrations to detect the segmentation. Xuhui et al. [34] propose a coarse liver segmentation using prior models for the shape, appearance and contextual information of the liver. An AdaBoost voxel-based classifier creates a liver probability map that is augmented in the last step with freeform deformation with a gradient appearance model. Next, we describe and compare these methods according to the different characteristics.

The methods of [7, 12, 15] are based on the registration to an atlas while the methods of [32, 34] require registration to a statistical shape model. Registration requires a presegmented dataset and is a time-consuming process and subject to inaccuracies. Only our work obviates the need for costly registration.

Most of the methods, including [12, 15, 32, 34] and our method, are based on a hierarchical process—organs are segmented in a predefined order to minimize segmentation errors and that of [7] segments all organs at once by image registration to a multiorgan atlas. We believe that hierarchical-based methods yield better results when compared to the method of [7] because they allow mutual information sharing between the segmentation processes of different organs.

While the VISCERAL Challenge is aimed at both enhanced and non-enhanced CT scans, our method is currently applicable only for enhanced CTs. Other methods are also applicable for non-enhanced CTs, thanks to the use of atlas/shape information. Currently, we are working on adapting our approach for non-enhanced CTs as well.

9.6   Conclusion

We have presented a new fully automatic atlas-free segmentation method of multiple organs of the ventral cavity in CT scans. Our method is unique in that it obviates the need for a predefined atlas and/or costly registration and in that it uses the same generic segmentation approach for all organs. Experimental results on 20 CECT scans of the VISCERAL Anatomy2 training dataset and 10 CECT scans of the Anatomy2 test dataset yield an average DICE volume overlap similarity score of 90.95 and 88.50%, respectively.

Automatic segmentation of anatomical structures in CT scans is an essential step in the analysis of radiological patient data and is a prerequisite for large-scale content-based image retrieval (CBIR) systems. Worldwide, the number of volumetric medical images (CT, MRI, etc.) reaches into the hundreds of millions per year and represents the largest single component of the medical health record. This untapped gold mine of medical data awaits the application of big data analytics, such as CBIR, to enable large-scale population and epidemiological studies, preventive medicine by early detection and assist radiologists in the decision-making process. The cloud-based evaluation framework of the VISCERAL Benchmarks [14] required source code to be submitted for testing by the organizers, the code was independently tested and we published it online[2]—it is now freely available for the benefit of the CBIR community. Future work consists of extending our approach to additional imaging modalities such as non-enhanced CT, handling scans of patients with organs missing, and testing the applicability of our method in an end-to-end CBIR scheme.

References

1. Aljabar P, Heckemann RA, Hammers A, Hajnal JV, Rueckert D (2009) Multi-atlas based segmentation of brain images: atlas selection and its effect on accuracy. NeuroImage 46(3):726–738
2. Boykov Y, Funka-Lea G (2006) Graph cuts and efficient N-D image segmentation. Int J Comput Vis 70(2):109–131
3. Caselles V, Kimmel R, Sapiro G (1997) Geodesic active contours. Int J Comput Vis 22(1):61–79
4. Deserno TM, Antani S, Long R (2009) Ontology of gaps in content-based image retrieval. J Digit Imaging 22(2):202–215
5. Freiman M, Eliassaf O, Taieb Y, Joskowicz L, Azraq Y, Sosna J (2008) An iterative bayesian approach for nearly automatic liver segmentation: algorithm and validation. Int J Comput Assist Radiol Surg 3(5):439–446
6. Freiman M, Kronman A, Esses SJ, Joskowicz L, Sosna J (2010) Non-parametric iterative model constraint graph min-cut for automatic kidney segmentation. Med Image Comput Comput Assist Interv, 13:73–80
7. Goksel O, Gass T, Szekely G (2014) Segmentation and landmark localization based on multiple atlases. In: CEUR workshop proceedings, pp 37–43
8. Gudewar AD, Ragha LR (2012) Ontology to improve CBIR system. Int J Comput Appl 52(21):23–30
9. Haris K, Efstratiadis SN, Maglaveras N, Katsaggelos AK (1998) Hybrid image segmentation using watershed and fast region merging. IEEE Trans Image Process 7(12):1684–1699
10. Heimann T, Meinzer HP (2009) Statistical shape models for 3D medical image segmentation: a review. Med Image Anal 13(4):543–563
11. Hwang KH, Lee H, Choi D (2012) Medical image retrieval: past and present. Healthc Inf Res 18(1):3–9
12. Jiménez del Toro ÓA, Müller H (2014) Multi-structure atlas-based segmentation using anatomical regions of interest. In: Menze B, Langs G, Montillo A, Kelm M, Müller H, Tu Z (eds) MCV 2013. LNCS, vol 8331. Springer, Cham, pp 217–221. doi:10.1007/978-3-319-05530-5_21
13. Jiménez del Toro OA, Goksel O, Menze B, Müller H, Langs G, Weber MA, Eggel I, Gruenberg K, Holzer M, Jakab A, Kotsios-Kontokotsios G, Krenn M, Fernandez TS, Schaer R, Taha AA, Winterstein M, Hanbury A (2014) VISCERAL—VISual concept extraction challenge in RAdioLogy: ISBI 2014 challenge organization. In: Goksel O (ed) Proceedings of the VISCERAL challenge at ISBI, Beijing, China, no. 1194 in CEUR workshop proceedings, pp 6–15. http://ceur-ws.org/Vol-1194/visceralISBI14-0.pdf

---

[2]http://www.cs.huji.ac.il/~caslab.

14. Jiménez del Toro OA, Müller H, Krenn M, Gruenberg K, Taha AA, Winterstein M, Eggel I, Foncubierta-Rodriguez A, Goksel O, Jakab A, Kontokotsios G, Langs G, Menze B, Fernandez TS, Schaer R, Walleyo A, Weber MA, Cid YD, Gass T, Heinrich M, Jia F, Kahl F, Kechichian R, Mai D, Spanier A, Vincent G, Wang C, Wyeth D, Hanbury A (2016) Cloud-based evaluation of anatomical structure segmentation and landmark detection algorithms: visceral anatomy benchmarks. IEEE Trans Med Imaging 99:1–1. doi:10.1109/TMI.2016.2578680

15. Kéchichian R, Valette S, Sdika M, Desvignes M (2014) Automatic 3D multiorgan segmentation via clustering and graph cut using spatial relations and hierarchically-registered atlases. In: Menze B, Langs G, Montillo A, Kelm M, Müller H, Zhang S, Cai WT, Metaxas D (eds) MCV 2014. LNCS, vol 8848. Springer, Cham, pp 201–209. doi:10.1007/978-3-319-13972-2_19

16. Kronman A, Joskowicz L, Sosna J (2012) Anatomical structures segmentation by spherical 3D ray casting and gradient domain editing. In: Ayache N, Delingette H, Golland P, Mori K (eds) MICCAI 2012. LNCS, vol 7511. Springer, Heidelberg, pp 363–370. doi:10.1007/978-3-642-33418-4_45

17. Langs G, Hanbury A, Menze B, Müller H (2013) VISCERAL: towards large data in medical imaging — challenges and directions. In: Greenspan H, Müller H, Syeda-Mahmood T (eds) MCBR-CDS 2012. LNCS, vol 7723. Springer, Heidelberg, pp 92–98. doi:10.1007/978-3-642-36678-9_9

18. Mharib AM, Rahman A, Mashohor S, Binti R (2012) Survey on liver CT image segmentation methods. Artif Intell Rev 37(2):83–95

19. Müller H, Zhou X, Depeursinge A, Pitkanen M, Iavindrasana J, Geissbuhler A (2007) Medical visual information retrieval: state of the art and challenges ahead. In: IEEE international conference on multimedia and expo. IEEE, pp 683–686

20. Ng AY, Jordan MI, Weiss Y (2002) On spectral clustering: analysis and an algorithm. Adv Neural Inf Process Syst 2:849–856

21. Okada T, Yokota K, Hori M, Nakamoto M, Nakamura H, Sato Y (2008) Construction of hierarchical multi-organ statistical atlases and their application to multi-organ segmentation from CT images. In: Metaxas D, Axel L, Fichtinger G, Székely G (eds) MICCAI 2008. LNCS, vol 5241. Springer, Heidelberg, pp 502–509. doi:10.1007/978-3-540-85988-8_60

22. Pham DL, Xu C, Prince JL (2000) Current methods in medical image segmentation. Annu Rev Biomed Eng 2(1):315–337

23. Rohlfing T, Brandt R, Menzel R, Russakoff DB, Maurer CR (2005) Quo vadis, atlas-based segmentation? Springer, Boston

24. Rubin DL (2011) Informatics in radiology: measuring and improving quality in radiology: meeting the challenge with informatics. Radiographics 31(6):1511–1527

25. Rubin DL (2012) Finding the meaning in images: annotation and image markup (maintained). Philos Psychiatry Psychol 18(4):311–318

26. Schmidt G, Athelogou M (2007) Cognition network technology for a fully automated 3D segmentation of liver. In: Proceedings of the MICCAI workshop 3-D segmentation clinic: a grand, challenge, pp 125–133

27. Simonyan K, Zisserman A, Criminisi A (2011) Immediate structured visual search for medical images. In: Fichtinger G, Martel A, Peters T (eds) MICCAI 2011. LNCS, vol 6893. Springer, Heidelberg, pp 288–296. doi:10.1007/978-3-642-23626-6_36

28. Sluimer I, Schilham A, Prokop M, van Ginneken B (2006) Computer analysis of computed tomography scans of the lung: a survey. IEEE Trans Med Imaging 25:385–405

29. Tong T, Wolz R, Wang Z, Gao Q, Misawa K, Fujiwara M, Mori K, Hajnal JV, Rueckert D (2015) Discriminative dictionary learning for abdominal multi-organ segmentation. Med Image Anal 23(1):92–104

30. Tsai A, Yezzi A Jr, Wells W, Tempany C, Tucker D, Fan A, Grimson WE, Willsky A (2003) A shape-based approach to the segmentation of medical imagery using level sets. Med Imaging 22(2):137–154

31. Valente F, Costa C, Silva A (2013) Content based retrieval systems in a clinical context, chap 1. In: Felix Erondu O (ed) Medical imaging in clinical practice. InTech, Rijeka

32. Wang C, Smedby O (2014) Automatic multi-organ segmentation in non-enhanced CT datasets using hierarchical shape priors. In: 22nd international conference on pattern recognition (ICPR), pp 3327–3332
33. Wolz R, Chu C, Misawa K, Mori K, Rueckert D (2012) Multi-organ abdominal CT segmentation using hierarchically weighted subject-specific atlases. In: Ayache N, Delingette H, Golland P, Mori K (eds) MICCAI 2012. LNCS, vol 7510. Springer, Heidelberg, pp 10–17. doi:10.1007/978-3-642-33415-3_2
34. Li X, Huang C, Jia F, Li Z, Fang C, Fan Y (2014) Automatic liver segmentation using statistical prior models and free-form deformation. In: Menze B, Langs G, Montillo A, Kelm M, Müller H, Zhang S, Cai WT, Metaxas D (eds) MCV 2014. LNCS, vol 8848. Springer, Cham, pp 181–188. doi:10.1007/978-3-319-13972-2_17

Chapter 10
Multiorgan Segmentation Using Coherent Propagating Level Set Method Guided by Hierarchical Shape Priors and Local Phase Information

Chunliang Wang and Örjan Smedby

Abstract In this chapter, we introduce an automatic multiorgan segmentation method using a hierarchical-shape-prior-guided level set method. The hierarchical shape priors are organized according to the anatomical hierarchy of the human body, so that the children structures are always contained by the parent structure. This hierarchical approach solves two challenges of multiorgan segmentation. First, it gradually refines the prediction of the organs' position by locating and segmenting the larger parent structure. Second, it solves the ambiguity of boundary between two attaching organs by looking at a large scale and imposing the additional shape constraint of the higher-level structures. To improve the segmentation accuracy, a model-guided local phase term is introduced and integrated with the conventional region-based energy function to guide the level set propagation. Finally, a novel coherent propagation method is implemented to speed up the model-based level set segmentation. In the VISCERAL Anatomy challenge, the proposed method delivered promising results on a number of abdominal organs.

C. Wang (✉) · Ö. Smedby
Center for Medical Image Science and Visualization (CMIV), Linköping University, Linköping, Sweden
e-mail: chunliang.wang@liu.se

Ö. Smedby
e-mail: orjan.smedby@sth.kth.se

C. Wang · Ö. Smedby
Department of Radiology and Department of Medical and Health Sciences, Linköping University, Linköping, Sweden

C. Wang · Ö. Smedby
School of Technology and Health (STH), KTH Royal Institute of Technology, Stockholm, Sweden

© The Author(s) 2017
A. Hanbury et al. (eds.), *Cloud-Based Benchmarking of Medical Image Analysis*, DOI 10.1007/978-3-319-49644-3_10

10.1   Introduction

Shape-prior-guided image segmentation methods are popular choices for various challenging segmentation tasks [4, 5, 7, 13, 18]. This is because the constraint from shape priors substantially reduces the risk of region leaking that could occur often if the segmentation algorithm merely relies on image features. However, in our experience, this constraint is no guarantee for successful segmentation, as undesired segmentation errors can still occur due to non-ideal model initialization or weak organ edge discrimination, which often happens when two neighbouring organs have similar intensity. Figure 10.1b shows an example of such failed shape-prior-guided segmentation. In this non-contrast CT scan, the liver model is misled towards the heart and chest wall by the similar intensity of these organs and the lack of gradient at the organ boundaries. This error could potentially be corrected if the segmentation algorithm incorporates some more sophisticated edge filters/detectors to enhance the vague borders between organs [9, 25]. However, such efforts often result in unstable solutions that will only work for a certain type of image and are sensitive to image quality and intensity variations. On the other hand, when asking a medical expert to perform the same task, such "absurd" errors will never happen, as the human observer has already identified the heart area and chest wall using his/her anatomical knowledge. In other words, the expert is doing a multiorgan segmentation even when he/she is asked to perform a single-organ segmentation. This led us to a simple philosophy: when it is difficult to tell whether a voxel belongs to organ A or not, it is probably easier to check whether it belongs to organ B or C. Based on this philosophy and the hierarchical nature of the human anatomy, we developed a hierarchical-shape-prior-guided multiorgan segmentation method. In the hierarchical shape model, the major structures with less population variation are at the top and smaller structures

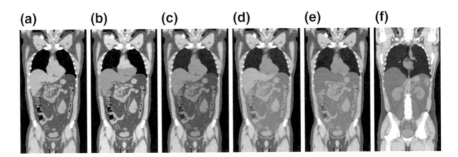

(a)   **(b)**   **(c)**   **(d)**   **(e)**   **(f)**

Fig. 10.1 A comparison between the conventional single-organ segmentation method (**b**) and the proposed hierarchical multiorgan approach (**c–f**). **a** Coronal view of a non-enhanced CT scan (note that the intensities of the liver, chest wall and heart are almost identical). **b** Failed liver segmentation with a single-organ shape prior. **c** Shape-prior-based ventral cavity segmentation. **d** Abdominopelvic cavity segmentation (*yellow*) on top of the ventral cavity (*red*). **e** Liver segmentation (*brown*) on *top* of ventral and abdominopelvic cavity segmentation. **f** Final multiorgan segmentation result. (Images are from our previous publication [17])

with higher irregularities are linked at a lower level. As shown in Fig. 10.1c–e, the segmentation starts from a large scale, so that the border between the ventral cavity and the chest and abdominal wall (Fig. 10.1c) is delineated, and then, at a smaller scale the, border between the thoracic and abdominal cavity (Fig. 10.1d) is identified. At the finest scale, individual organs are segmented (Fig. 10.1e).

The proposed top-down approach solves two major challenges of organ segmentation. The first one is to locate the anatomical structures within the dataset. Due to respiratory motion and anatomical variation, even for the scans with similar scanning range, the location of the same organ can still vary considerably. In the proposed multiorgan segmentation framework, the location information of the major structures is first detected with higher confidence and then passed down to the lower-level structures to initialize their segmentation. This process is similar to a multi-resolution registration approach. However, the benefit of using statistical shape models at each level is that the negative influence of anatomical and appearance variation of finer structures is eliminated to a large extent. The other major challenge that the proposed method solves is to delineate the boundary between two closely attached organs. Such delineation can be difficult in certain places where the contrast between organs is very vague or vanishes. In addition to the local features, the proposed method also utilizes the shape information of larger structures to guide the segmentation, i.e. the boundary information from higher-level structures provides extra cues to guide the segmentation of the lower-level structures. Such a hierarchical framework has proved to be very robust and performed relatively well even on non-contrast-enhanced CT image when using only region-based energy based on image intensity [16, 17].

To further improve the segmentation accuracy of the hierarchical model-based method, a model-guided edge-based energy term is proposed and combined with the region-based energy term to guide the level set evolution [19]. Unlike the conventional edge-based energy terms, which ignore the orientation of the edge-related features, the model-guided edge-based energy term uses the normal direction of the shape model to suggest the searching orientation of the local structures. This makes it possible to distinguish the black-to-white edges from white-to-black edges, which generate the same edge responses when using conventional gradient and local phase measurements. As such ambiguity often exists in the area where two organs' borders approach each other, there is a greater chance for the segmentation region to leak to the nearby organ when using conventional edge-based energy terms.

Finally, to improve segmentation speed, a novel coherent propagating level set algorithm was implemented. The new algorithm forces the contour to move monotonically according to a predicted developing trend which makes the level set functions converge faster. It also makes it possible to detect local convergence, so that the parts of the boundary that have reached their final position can be excluded in subsequent iterations, thus significantly reducing computation time [20, 22]. The proposed method was tested using the VISCERAL benchmark database, and promising results were delivered within reasonable processing time without any user intervention.

10.2 Statistical Shape-Prior-Guided Level Set Segmentation

As a member of the active contour family, the level set method segments the targeted object in an image by propagating an initial contour towards the object's border. The movement of the contour is usually guided by two types of forces: the external and internal forces. While the external force is often designed to drive the contour towards the object's border, the internal force is commonly designed to keep the contour smooth. To generate these forces, the segmentation problem is often formulated as an energy minimization problem, as demonstrated in Eq. 10.1, where ϕ is the level set function, and α, β are weighting factors.

$$E(\phi) = \alpha E_{in}(\phi) + \beta E_{ex}(\phi) \tag{10.1}$$

The most common external energy functions include region-based image energy and gradient-based image energy; examples are given in Eqs. 10.2 and 10.3, respectively. The former converts the input image intensity into probability functions of a pixel/voxel belonging to the object or the background [3], while the latter utilizes the image gradient to guide the movement of the contour so that the contour is attracted to areas with higher gradient [2].

$$E_{region}(\phi) = -\int \log\left[p_A(I(x))\right] H(\phi(x))\, dx - \int \log\left[p_B(I(x))\right] (1 - H(\phi(x)))\, dx \tag{10.2}$$

$$E_{edge}(\phi) = \int (|\nabla I(x)| + 1)^{-1} \phi'(x)\, dx \tag{10.3}$$

$$E_{in}(\phi) = \int |\nabla H(\phi(x))|\, dx \tag{10.4}$$

Here, H is the Heaviside function, and p_A and p_B are probability functions of a pixel belonging to the object region and the background region, respectively. The internal energy is often connected with local curvature of the contour, which means it is minimized when the contour becomes smooth (e.g. Eq. 10.4). The local smoothness character of active contours makes them resistant to noise. The internal force can also, to some extent, prevent the segmentation region leaking to a neighbouring object through small "holes" that connect two regions with similar appearance. However, as the curvature is a local measurement, if the connecting "holes" are larger than the scale at which the smoothness is measured, leaking problems may still occur. To obtain the right segmentation results in such cases, we need to impose a stronger constraint on the shape of the contour. While there is no general solution to avoid the leaking problem for all cases, in medical images, we can often use the prior knowledge of the anatomical shape of the targeted structures. The statistical shape model-guided level set method proposed by Leventon et al. is an example of incorporating such shape prior knowledge into the image segmentation [13]. In this framework, a shape-based energy term is added to penalize the differences between the evolving contour and the shape prior (Eq. 10.5):

$$E_{mode}(\phi) = \int (\phi(x) - m(t(x)))^2 \, dx \tag{10.5}$$

where m represents the statistical shape model, and t is a rigid transformation function.

How to represent the shape prior knowledge using mathematical models is still an active research field; a relatively complete review can be found in [5, 7]. In general, there are two types of statistical shape models that are commonly used for medical image segmentation. One is the mesh-based representations, such as the active shape models (ASMs) [4], where shapes are expressed as 2D contours or 3D meshes, and the variation of shapes is constrained by the distribution of the vertexes. Another type of shape models is region-based where the shapes are embedded in distance maps created from binary patterns. The latter is often used in the level set-based framework, since the level set function itself is also a distance map. For the mesh-based representations, it is less straightforward to define a transform function t relating the meshes with the level set function. To create the region-based statistical model, manually created segmentation masks are first aligned using rigid registration; i.e., only translation, rotation and isotropic scaling are allowed. Then, these aligned binary masks are converted into signed distance maps via a distance transform. The prominent variations of these distance maps can be obtained via principal component analysis (PCA). Finally, the statistical model is represented by combining the mean of the signed distance maps ($\overline{m}$) and a weighted combination of the variation maps ($m_{\sigma 1}, m_{\sigma 2}, \ldots m_{\sigma n}$) (Eq. 10.6).

$$M = \overline{m} + \omega_1 m_{\sigma 1} + \omega_2 m_{\sigma 2} + \cdots + \omega_n m_{\sigma n} \tag{10.6}$$

It should be pointed out that the PCA process mentioned above does not guarantee the algorithm to fully recover the population variation of the targeted shape. This is because the distance transform is a nonlinear process. It has been shown that in some cases, the shape variation is highly nonlinear [5]. This limits these types of methods to shapes that do not vary in a too complicated manner. Fortunately, this is often not a big problem for anatomical structures in medical applications.

Combining the region-based term and the model-based term as the external energy leads us to the level set equation minimizing Eq. 10.1:

$$\frac{\partial \phi}{\partial t} = \left[\alpha \, \text{div} \left(\frac{\nabla \phi}{|\nabla \phi|} \right) + \beta \left(\log(p_B) - \log(p_A) \right) + \gamma m(t) \right] |\nabla \phi| \tag{10.7}$$

The optimization of the level set function and the model fitting is usually performed iteratively in parallel; i.e., the model is re-estimated after one or several iterations of the level set evolution. The transformation t and the weighting factors

ω_i are usually solved by minimizing the squared distance between the model and the level set function, which is also a signed distance map.

10.3 Multiorgan Segmentation Using Hierarchical Shape Priors

Although using shape priors prevents the leaking problem in many medical application, in some challenging cases, a single-organ model is still insufficient to generate a satisfactory segmentation result. Such failure can often be seen in cases where the connecting area between two organs of similar intensity is relatively large. An example is given in Fig. 10.1b. In this non-enhanced CT scan, the liver model was confused by the similar intensity between the liver and other surrounding organs. Even though there are visible gaps between them, such small local minima cannot prevent the model-based segmentation method to reach a global minimum when minimizing Eq. 10.1. While the connecting areas are relatively large for the liver, they become smaller when looking at a higher scale. For example, when looking at the ventral cavity (union of thoracic cavity and abdominopelvic cavity), there is no longer ambiguity of telling which is the chest wall and which is the liver (Fig. 10.1c). It is the same for the border between the heart and the liver when looking at the separation of the thoracic and abdominal cavity (Fig. 10.1d). Therefore, it is advantageous to use hierarchical shape priors that are organized according to the scale and shape complexity of different anatomical structures; i.e., the large organs of more regular shape with less interobject variation are located at the higher level, and the smaller structures of more complex appearance and variation are introduced at a lower level. During the segmentation, higher-level structures' location information will influence the lower-level structures' location, and the higher-level structures' border will also limit the area of the lower-level structures as the latter are assumed to be contained by their upper-level structures.

10.3.1 Building Hierarchical Shape Priors

The major structures of the proposed hierarchical shape priors are listed in Fig. 10.2. Building hierarchical shape priors consists of two major steps: building individual shape models and linking them together in a common space. The individual statistical shape model generation is not much different from the traditional statistical shape generation process described in Sect. 10.2. However, to make sure that the relative scale between different structures is preserved, a "standard patient" is selected in the beginning via a visual comparison. Organs that are manually segmented from other patients are all registered towards the corresponding organ of this standard patient.

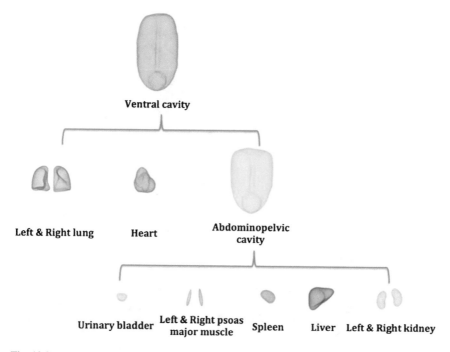

Fig. 10.2 An overview of the hierarchical organization of the shape priors

To link different organs and structures to a common space, the children-level struc-tures are projected into their parent-level structure's space using the transformation matrices that align the upper-level structures. For example, after the ventral cavity masks of all other subjects are registered towards the picked subject's ventral cavity, the children-level structures of those subjects, i.e. lungs, heart and abdominopelvic cavity, are projected to the mean shape of the ventral cavity using the same rigid transform as the ventral cavities. These structures will not be perfectly aligned, but the sum of the masks will form a probability map that suggests the likelihood of the corresponding organ appearing at a certain place of the ventral cavity. A binary trust zone of the lower-level organ is created by setting a threshold on the probability map. Finally, the mean shapes of these children structures are registered towards the corresponding trust zones. Through these chains of transformation, we establish a rigid transform from the mean shape of a children structure to its parent structure. These transformation matrices are used to initialize the position of the children struc-ture models, once the segmentation of their parent structures is finished. Figure 10.3 shows the mean shapes of all structures used in our hierarchical shape model and their relative positions determined using the approach describe here.

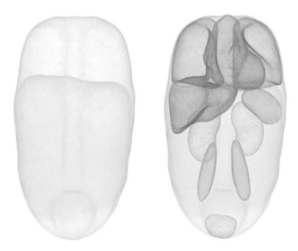

Fig. 10.3 The mean shape of different anatomical structures and their relative positions

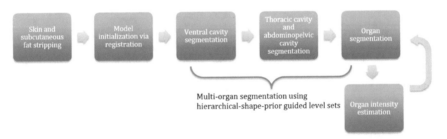

Fig. 10.4 The processing pipeline of the proposed multiorgan segmentation framework

10.3.2 Multiorgan Segmentation Using Hierarchical Shape Priors

Figure 10.4 summarizes the processing pipeline of the proposed segmentation framework. In a preprocessing step, we try to remove the skin and subcutaneous fat from the patient's image data using a threshold-based level set method combined with mathematical morphological operations. Because these tissues vary considerably from patient to patient, if present, they may mislead the following registration between the unseen patient and the standard patient mentioned above. This registration step is designed to initialize the ventral cavity model's position in the unseen patient. The segmentation steps are performed in a top-down fashion guided by the hierarchical shape model; i.e., the ventral cavity is first segmented and then divided into thoracic cavity and abdominopelvic cavity. At a third stage, the individual organs such as liver, spleen and kidneys are segmented. Within the same level, structures are segmented sequentially from left to right in the order listed in Fig. 10.2.

The segmentation process for individual structures is very similar to the model-guided level set method described in Sect. 10.2, except that an additional energy term is added to let the parent structure regulate the children structures' segmentation. The new energy function is given in Eq. 10.8.

$$E_{parent\_mode}(\phi) = \int \left(1 - H\left(\phi_p(x)\right) - H(\phi(x))\right)^2 dx \qquad (10.8)$$

Here, ϕ_p is the segmentation result of the parent structure. For the ventral cavity, ϕ_p is set to be the level set function of the subcutaneous fat stripping step. Note that as long as the children structure is inside its parent, the latter has no influence on the lower-level structure segmentation. Besides this regulation force, the segmentation of the parent structure also provides the initial position of the children structures using the relative transformation matrix obtained in the hierarchical shape model training phase.

10.3.3 Region-Based External Speed Function

Besides the model terms, the image term of the level set function is another important factor of the multiorgan framework. As presented in Sect. 10.2, common external speed functions include region-based methods and gradient-based methods. In our preliminary implementation of the proposed hierarchical-shape-prior-guided level set framework, we chose to use the region-based approach, where the external speed function is an intensity mapping function. Like the threshold-based level set method proposed by Lefohn et al. [12], the mapping function outputs a positive speed if the CT value is close to the mean intensity of a selected organ, but a negative speed when the CT value is unlikely to be seen in that organ. For non-contrast-enhanced CT scans, the intensity distribution of most parenchymal organs is relatively consistent from patient to patient, which allows us to use the same sets of parameters to guide the segmentation of the same organ in different subjects. Some examples are plotted in Fig. 10.5. Note that as the intensity distribution of some neighbouring organs/structures may overlap with the targeted organ, the ceiling and floor of the mapping function are manually tuned to avoid leaking into the neighbouring structures. This results in an asymmetric intensity mapping function, like for the ventral cavity. For contrast-enhanced CT scans, the intensity distribution of some organs may vary significantly depending on the circulation rate and acquisition timing, and an iterative intensity range estimation approach is then used for segmenting the heart, liver, kidney and spleen. Using the imperfect initial segmentation, we estimate the mean intensity (M) and its standard deviation (σ) of the targeted organ. The organ's upper and lower thresholds are then set to be $M + 1.5\sigma$ and $M - 1.5\sigma$, respectively. To avoid the influence of undesired tissue included in these preliminary segmentations, all voxels with intensity lower than 30HU are excluded from the calculation

Fig. 10.5 Example
thresholding functions for
the image term

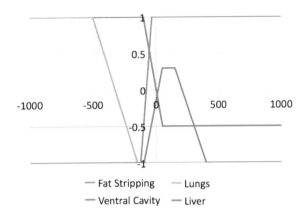

of M and σ. The intensity estimation is repeated during the model fitting process. The iterative intensity estimation stops when the changing rates of M and σ are both lower than a threshold (5 HU).

10.4 Improving Segmentation Accuracy Using Model-Guided Local Phase Analysis

Although the region-based speed function alone can generate relatively good segmentation results, in complicated cases where the organ is attached to several neighbouring structures with various intensity ranges, it is advantageous to rely not only on the image intensity but also on the edge information. Therefore, combining the region-based and gradient-based speed function is a natural way to improve the segmentation accuracy. However, conventional gradient-based edge delineation cannot distinguish between black-to-white and white-to-black edges. In medical images, we often see two organs approaching each other in some areas. As both edges generate high gradient measurements, the contour may be attracted to either side depending on the initial position of the contour. To avoid such ambiguity, we have proposed a model-guided local phase analysis that is able to distinguish between these two types of edges and avoid the segmentation region leaking into another organ.

10.4.1 Quadrature Filters and Model-Guided Local Phase Analysis

So-called quadrature filters are pairs of filters designed to measure whether the underlying image structure is similar to a ridge-like pattern or an edge-like pattern. An example of a two-dimensional quadrature pair set is shown in Fig. 10.6a, b. The

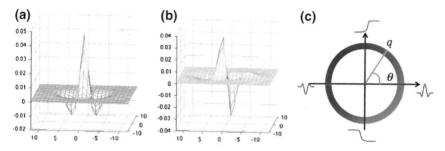

Fig. 10.6   An example of quadrature filter pairs in 2D. **a** The ridge-picking filter. **b** The edge-picking filter. **c** The quadrature filter's response in the complex plane

output of this pair of filters is represented by a complex number where the real part is the output of the ridge-picking filter and the imaginary part is the output of the edge-picking filter. The argument of this complex number in the complex plane is referred to as the *local phase* [10], θ in Fig. 10.6c. The magnitude (q) of the complex number is called *local energy* [10]. Local phase is often used as a promising alternative to image gradient for image segmentation [1, 11, 18]. This is because the phase measure measurement changes monotonically when moving from one side of the edge to the other side, which makes it easier to design a speed function. However, like gradient measurements, local phase is also orientation-dependent. In practice, the local phase is often estimated using the local orientation estimated from the local gradient or eigenvectors of the local structure tensor. These types of solutions will produce the same phase for black-to-white and white-to-black edges. When used for segmentation, the local phase still cannot prevent the contour from leaking to the edge of a neighbouring organ.

Here, we propose to use the evolving statistical shape model, instead of the input image, to generate the reference direction for local phase measurement. This is done by converting the shape model into a signed distance map. When measuring the local phase at a point, the principle orientation of the quadrature filters is then aligned with the gradient of the signed distance map. Note that the reference orientation is perpendicular to the shape surface. More importantly, the gradient also indicates which direction is inside and outside. Unlike conventional local phase analysis, the output of the model-based phase analysis is $\pi/2$ on a black-to-white edge and $-\pi/2$ on a white-to-black edge. An example of applying the proposed phase analysis in a brain MRI volume is shown in Fig. 10.7h. Compared with the phase map produced by Läthén's method [11] (Fig. 10.7d), the proposed solution (Fig. 10.2h) makes a clear distinction between the inner boundary of the skull (blue) and the outer surface of the brain (yellow).

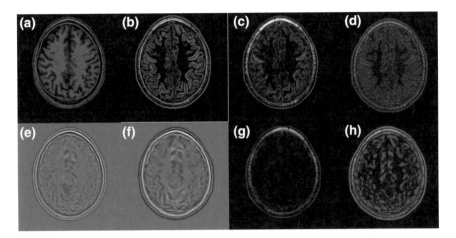

Fig. 10.7 **a** Input image: the *green* contour represents the cross section of the brain model; **b** the gradient magnitude; **c, d** local energy and phase maps using Läthén's method [11]; **e, f, g, h** the real and imaginary parts of the model-guided quadrature filter and corresponding local energy and phase maps. (**d, h** were created using the colour lookup table shown in Fig. 10.6c)

10.4.2 Integrating Region-Based and Edge-Based Energy in the Level Set Method

To use the phase information to guide the level set propagation, we propose an energy function as described in Eq. 10.9.

$$E(\partial\mathcal{R}) = \int_0^1 g\left[\theta\left(I\left(\partial\mathcal{R}_A(c)\right)\right) - \tau\right]^2 |\mathcal{R}_A(c)| \, dc \qquad (10.9)$$

Here, I is the input image, $\mathcal{R}_A$ is the segmented region, and θ is the estimated local phase $(0 \leq \theta < 2\pi)$ at any given location. τ is the targeted phase (e.g. $\pi/2$ for a black-to-white edge and $3\pi/2$ for a white-to-black edge). The function g is simply a period-fixing function that ensures that the phase difference $\theta - \tau$ falls in the range from $-\pi$ to π (Eq. 10.10).

$$g(\delta) = \begin{cases} \delta & \text{if } -\pi < \delta \leq \pi \\ \delta - 2\pi & \text{if } \delta > \pi \\ \delta + 2\pi & \text{if } \delta \leq -\pi \end{cases} \qquad (10.10)$$

Note that Eq. 10.9 is very similar to the conventional geodesic active contours given in Eq. 10.3, except that $\theta(I)$ replaces ∇I, and the period-fixing function g replaces the gradient magnitude inverse function. To combine the phase-based energy and the region-based energy, we propose an integrated energy function:

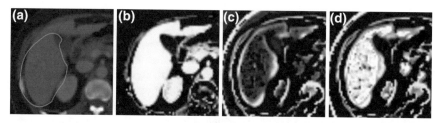

Fig. 10.8 **a** An axial view of an input volume (*green* contour shows the current shape model), (**b**) the region-based speed terms based on the image intensity, **c** the phase-based term estimated using the model, **d** the combined external speed map. Note that the connection between liver and kidney is removed

$$E\left(\partial\mathscr{R}\right) = \alpha \int_0^1 g\left[\theta\left(I\left(\partial\mathscr{R}_A\left(c\right)\right)\right) - \tau\right]^2 \left|\mathscr{R}_A\left(c\right)\right| dc -$$
$$\int_{\mathscr{R}_A} \int w(x,y)\log\left[p_A\left(I\left(x,y\right)\right)\right]dxdy \; - \int_{\mathscr{R}_B}\int w(x,y)\log\left[p_B\left(I\left(x,y\right)\right)\right]dxdy$$

$$(10.11)$$

Here, p_A and p_B are the probability functions of a given pixel/voxel belonging to the region A/B. Function w is a weighting function that weights the fitting energy using the local energy output (q) from the quadrature filter, as described in Eq. 10.12:

$$w(x,y) = \frac{1}{1 + q\left(I\left(x,y\right)\right)}$$

$$(10.12)$$

The energy function is minimized by solving the following descent equation:

$$\frac{\partial\phi}{\partial t} = \left[\alpha g(\theta - \tau)^2 \mathrm{div}\left(\frac{\nabla\phi}{|\nabla\phi|}\right) + \alpha g(\theta - \tau) + w\log(p_B) - w\log(p_A) + m(t)\right]|\nabla\phi|$$

$$(10.13)$$

Figure 10.8 shows an example of integrated speed in a liver segmentation case. The region-based and phase-based components of the speed function are also shown side by side. In practice, the first component on the right side can be replaced by $\alpha'\mathrm{div}\left(\frac{\nabla\phi}{|\nabla\phi|}\right)$, where α' is a weighting factor, as it is just a regulation term that corresponds to the curvature force in the conventional level set methods.

Since the filter orientation varies across the image, the filtering is made via local resampling by rotating a given kernel grid to align with the local reference direction. This step can also be carried out using a steerable filter, which synthesizes a filter with arbitrary orientation from a linear combination of basis filters [6]. The latter may be faster if the local phase analysis needs to be performed for all pixels/voxels. However, in practice, the computation on points that are far away from the model surface can be skipped, as will be further explained in the next section.

10.5 Speeding up Level Set Segmentation Using Coherent Propagation

Level set methods are computationally intensive, and many efforts have been made to speed up level set-based segmentation. One common approach is to limit the computation to a narrow band around the zero level set. The most popular implementation of this type is the sparse field level set, which only updates the level set function on a 1-pixel wide band that the zero level set passes through [24]. However, the processing time is still in the range of 10–30 min to segment a single organ from a voxel image [22]. To speed up level set segmentation, we proposed a fast level set method using coherent propagation [20, 22]. The new method not only limits the computation to a narrow band, but also eliminates the points that have reached the object border. This local convergence detection is enabled by synchronizing local points on the contour to move outwards or inwards together monotonically in a period instead of letting different points on a contour move outwards or inwards simultaneously. The speed function of the coherent propagating level set can be written as in Eq. 10.14.

$$\frac{\partial \phi}{\partial t} = W\left(V_t\right) \quad \text{where} \quad W\left(V_t\right) = \begin{cases} V_t\left(x\right) & \text{if } V_t\left(x\right) Tr\left(x\right) > 0 \\ 0 & \text{if } V_t\left(x\right) Tr\left(x\right) \leq 0 \end{cases} \quad (10.14)$$

Here, V_t is the conventional level set speed function (e.g. Eq. 10.7), and the function Tr represents a trend direction suggesting whether the local contour is expanding or shrinking. Within a single period, its value is fixed to 1 or -1. The initial value of Tr can be either estimated using the average external speed in a neighbourhood [22] or assigned via user interaction, such as dragging the contour inwards or outwards [23]. In the latter case, the trend of the whole contour is synchronized, meaning that the contour is designed to only expand or shrink in the first period. A period ends when no points on the contour can move towards the trend direction. When entering the next period, the Tr function will switch sign at all points, and all points will propagate in the opposite direction until they stop again. The final segmentation result can be obtained after repeating the coherent propagation for a small number of periods (4–6). Within a single period, once $W\left(x\right)$ returns 0, at point x, then this point is excluded from the further computation, until at least one of its neighbours' level set value has changed. The ability to detect the converged points helps the new level set method to achieve at least 10 times speedup in various segmentation tasks when compared with the sparse field level set algorithm [22].

Moving from level set segmentation to statistical shape model-guided level set segmentation, the computational burden becomes even greater. While simply plugging Eq. 10.7 as v_t into Eq. 10.14 can already speed up the segmentation process considerably, another time-consuming part of model-based level set segmentation is to update the statistical model iteratively as the level set propagates. Although the narrowband strategy can also be applied here, i.e. using the voxel on the zero level set to drive the statistical shape fitting, the computation can still be slow if the fitting has to be repeated frequently. To reduce the frequency of updating the shape model, we limit the maximum travel distance of the active contour from the previous shape model by normalizing the image terms in Eq. 10.3 and tuning the weighting factors. This maximum travel distance is often set to be relatively small (3–5 mm), which means that the model fitting need not be repeated before the level set converges. When using the conventional level set method, it is not possible to know when the level set function will converge, and the level set evolution is often repeated a redundant number of iterations, which may outweigh the benefit of reducing the number of registrations. On the other hand, the coherent propagation method is capable of detecting the convergence by itself, thereby avoiding such redundant computations. In our preliminary experience of the new framework, the model fitting rarely needs to be repeated more than 20 times, given a relatively good initialization. The reduced model updating frequency will also directly benefit the model-guided phase computation, which can be very time-consuming, too. Moreover, since the contour is not allowed to move further than the maximum travel distance, we only need to compute the local phase for the points on the narrow band.

10.6   Experiments and Results

The proposed method was tested for multiorgan segmentation using the data from the VISCERAL multiorgan segmentation Benchmark.[1] Our method was trained using 7 non-enhanced CT (CT) and 7 contrast-enhanced CT (CECT) datasets (the 14 training datasets from the VISCERAL Anatomy 1 challenge [8]) and tested on 8 non-enhanced and 10 enhanced CT datasets. In our experiments, we tested three implementations of the proposed method:

Implementation 1: Hierarchical model-guided multiorgan segmentation uses only the region-based speed function described in Sect. 10.3.3. The segmentation was made at a single resolution of 3 mm isotropic voxel size.

Implementation 2: Hierarchical model-guided multiorgan segmentation uses the combined local phase- and intensity-based speed function described in Sect. 10.4.2. The segmentation was done at a single resolution of 3 mm isotropic voxel size.

Implementation 3: Hierarchical model-guided multiorgan segmentation uses the combined local phase- and intensity-based speed function described in Sect. 10.4.2. The segmentation was done using a multi-resolution strategy, and the finest resolution was same as the input image.

Detailed results and comparison of these three implementations are listed in Table 10.1. We further tested the influence of two key parameters in the preprocessing step on the segmentation accuracy: the Gaussian smoothing kernel size and the downsample spacing. The results are plotted in Fig. 10.9. All these experiments were done using Implementation 1.

---

[1]VISCERAL   Benchmark,   http://www.visceral.eu/closed-benchmarks/anatomy2/anatomy2-results/.

Table 10.1 Multiorgan segmentation in CT and CECT datasets (mean Dice coefficient)

Data	Method	Liver	Right Kidney	Left Kidney	Spleen	Right Lung	Left Lung
CT (8 cases)	Implementation 1	93.3%	77.9%	87.6%	90.1%	96.0%	95.9%
	Implementation 2	93.2%	71.7%	88.8%	91.0%	96.3%	95.9%
	Implementation 3	93.6%	79.6%	89.6%	91.0%	97.0%	96.1%
CECT (10 cases)	Implementation 1	92.9%	92.2%	92.6%	87.0%	96.6%	96.6%
	Implementation 2	93.9%	92.2%	92.4%	88.9%	96.7%	96.7%
	Implementation 3	94.9%	95.9%	94.5%	90.9%	97.1%	97.2%

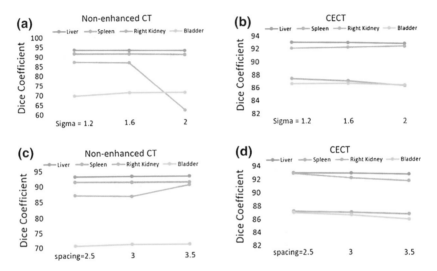

Fig. 10.9 **a, b** Plot of the segmentation accuracy measured with Dice coefficient against the size of the smoothing kernel (measured in voxels). **c, d** Plot of the segmentation accuracy against the image resolution used for the segmentation (measured in mm)

The average processing time for segmenting 10 selected organs was about 15 min for Implementation 1, 25 min for Implementation 2 and 55 min for Implementation 3, when running on a PC with Intel i7 (1.9 GHz). A $7 \times 7 \times 7$ quadrature filter with a central frequency of $\pi/2$ and a bandwidth of 6 octaves was used for the experiments.

10.7   Discussion and Conclusion

In the VISCERAL Anatomy Segmentation Benchmark [8], the proposed method outperformed conventional methods in terms of accuracy for brain stripping and liver, spleen and kidney segmentation tasks. Compared with other registration-based multi-atlas approaches that delivered superior results on some other structures [8], the proposed method has the advantage of being more computationally efficient. It is also interesting to note that some single-organ approaches fall behind the multiorgan approaches in terms of accuracy. This, to some extent, proves our hypothesis that it is easier to tell the membership of voxel in a multiorgan setup than looking at a single organ.

In our experience, image smoothing is an inevitable step for our method to be able to work on non-contrast-enhanced CT, as these images are very noisy. Using a large smoothing kernel may help the active contours to avoid stopping prematurely. However, when the organs' intensities are very similar, using a large smoothing kernel may destroy the vague edges between two organs and lead to total failure. This could partly explain the relatively random results plotted in Fig. 10.9a. When dealing with contrast-enhanced CT images with high signal-to-noise ratio (SNR), the smoothing kernel applied before the image segmentation in general has a negative effect on the segmentation accuracy.

The downsampling rate is another key parameter to consider when balancing the segmentation accuracy and the processing time. As suggested by Fig. 10.9d, higher downsampling rates often lead to worse segmentation results. This can also be seen when comparing the results from Implementation 1 and Implementation 2. However, for non-contrast-enhanced CT images, the downsampling itself will have some smoothing effect, and therefore, unpredicted sharp performance jumps/drops may be observed (e.g. Fig. 10.9c).

In this preliminary study, the training samples that were used to create the statistical shape models were arbitrarily chosen without carefully investigating the proper training sample selection strategy or variation enlarging methods mentioned in [7]. This is partly due to the fact that the current implementation of the training pipeline is not fully automated. Manual adjustment is involved in the registration and position linking steps. Although the segmentation results seem to be relatively accurate on the 18 testing datasets, we expect the results to degrade when applying the current shape models to a larger population. To implement a more sophisticated training sample selection strategy and build better statistical shape models using a larger training sample group have been planned.

So far, the proposed solution can only selectively segment 10 anatomical structures. While extending the current framework to segment more structures is relatively easy, it may not deliver satisfactory results for all of them. Two challenges are expected on some of the other smaller structures: great position variation and great shape variation. The proposed method relies on the initial position of the shape model being relatively close to the target organ. If the relative position of the parent structure is far from the child structure, the proposed method may, in extreme cases, miss the targeted organ entirely. We plan to solve this problem by introducing machine-learning-based organ detectors [14]. These detectors could also help us handle heterogeneous cases with varying scan ranges. On the other hand, the distance map-based statistical shape model used here may not be an ideal representation for all anatomical structures, in particular for those structures with high anatomical variation. Changing the statistical shape model to skeleton-based models may be more suitable for segmenting such structures, as suggested in [15, 21].

In conclusion, the hierarchical shape model-guided multiorgan segmentation method is a promising approach to solve the ambiguity between two attaching organs. By introducing a model-based local phase term into the energy function and solving the minimization problem using our novel coherent propagation algorithm, we have demonstrated that the proposed multiorgan segmentation method can deliver accurate results using relatively short processing times.

References

1. Belaid A, Boukerroui D, Maingourd Y, Lerallut JF (2011) Phase-based level set segmentation of ultrasound images. IEEE Trans Inf Technol Biomed 15(1):138–147. doi:10.1109/TITB. 2010.2090889
2. Caselles V, Kimmel R, Sapiro G (1997) Geodesic active contours. Int J Comput Vis 22(1):61–79. doi:10.1023/A:1007979827043
3. Chan TF, Vese LA (2001) Active contours without edges. IEEE Trans Image Process 10(2):266–277. doi:10.1109/83.902291
4. Cootes T, Taylor C, Cooper D, Graham J (1995) Active shape models-their training and application. Comput Vis Image Underst 61(1):38–59. doi:10.1006/cviu.1995.1004
5. Cremers D, Rousson M, Deriche R (2007) A review of statistical approaches to level set segmentation: integrating color, texture, motion and shape. Int J Comput Vis 72(2):195–215. doi:10.1007/s11263-006-8711-1
6. Freeman WT, Adelson EH (1991) The design and use of steerable filters. IEEE Trans Pattern Anal Mach Intell 13(9):891–906. doi:10.1109/34.93808
7. Heimann T, Meinzer HP (2009) Statistical shape models for 3D medical image segmentation: a review. Med Image Anal 13(4):543–563. doi:10.1016/j.media.2009.05.004
8. Jiménez del Toro OJ, Müller H, Krenn M, Gruenberg K, Taha AA, Winterstein M, Eggel I, Foncubierta-Rodriguez A, Goksel O, Jakab A, Kontokotsios G, Langs G, Menze B, Fernandez TS, Schaer R, Walleyo A, Weber MA, Cid YD, Gass T, Heinrich M, Jia F, Kahl F, Kechichian R, Mai D, Spanier A, Vincent G, Wang C, Wyeth D, Hanbury A (2016) Cloud-based evaluation of anatomical structure segmentation and landmark detection algorithms: VISCERAL anatomy benchmarks. IEEE Trans Med Imaging. doi:10.1109/TMI.2016.2578680
9. Kainmueller D, Lange T, Lamecker H (2007) Shape constrained automatic segmentation of the liver based on a heuristic intensity model. In: Proceedings of MICCAI workshop on 3D segmentation in the clinic: a grand challenge, pp 109–116
10. Knutsson H (1994) Signal processing for computer vision. Springer, Berlin
11. Läthén G, Jonasson J, Borga M (2010) Blood vessel segmentation using multi-scale quadrature filtering. Pattern Recognit Lett 31(8):762–767. doi:10.1016/j.patrec.2009.09.020
12. Lefohn AE, Cates JE, Whitaker RT (2003) Interactive, GPU-based level sets for 3D segmentation. In: Ellis RE, Peters TM (eds) Proceedings of the 6th international conference medical image computing and computer-assisted intervention—MICCAI, Montréal, Canada, Nov 15–18, 2003. Springer, Berlin, pp 564–572. doi:10.1007/978-3-540-39899-8_70
13. Leventon ME, Grimson WEL, Faugeras O (2000) Statistical shape influence in geodesic active contours. In: Proceedings of the IEEE conference on computer vision and pattern recognition, 2000, vol 1, pp 316–323. doi:10.1109/CVPR.2000.855835
14. Wang C, Lundström C (2016) CT scan range estimation using multiple body parts detection: let PACS learn the CT image content. Int J Comput Assist Radiol Surg 11(2):317–325. doi:10.1007/s11548-015-1232-z
15. Wang C, Smedby Ö (2013) Fully automatic brain segmentation using model-guided level sets and skeleton-based models. MIDAS J

16. Wang C, Smedby Ö (2014) Automatic multi-organ segmentation using fast model based level set method and hierarchical shape priors. In: Goksel O (ed) Proceedings of the VISCERAL challenge at ISBI, Beijing, China, no. 1194 in CEUR workshop proceedings, pp 25–31. http://ceur-ws.org/Vol-1194/visceralISBI14-0.pdf
17. Wang C, Smedby Ö (2014) Automatic multi-organ segmentation in non-enhanced CT datasets using hierarchical shape priors. In: 2014 22nd international conference on pattern recognition (ICPR), pp 3327–3332. doi:10.1109/ICPR.2014.574
18. Wang C, Smedby Ö (2014) Model-based left ventricle segmentation in 3D ultrasound using phase image. MIDAS J
19. Wang C, Smedby Ö (2015) Multi-organ segmentation using shape model guided local phase analysis. Springer, Berlin, pp 149–156. doi:10.1007/978-3-319-24574-4_18
20. Wang C, Frimmel H, Smedby O (2011) Level-set based vessel segmentation accelerated with periodic monotonic speed function. In: Proceedings of the SPIE medical imaging conference, p 79621M. doi:10.1117/12.876704
21. Wang C, Moreno R, Smedby Ö (2012) Vessel segmentation using implicit model-guided level sets. In: Proceedings of the 3D cardiovascular imaging: a MICCAI segmentation challenge workshop
22. Wang C, Frimmel H, Smedby O (2014) Fast level-set based image segmentation using coherent propagation. Med Phys 41(7):073501. doi:10.1118/1.4881315
23. Wang C, Dahlström N, Fransson SG, Lundström C, Smedby Ö (2015) Real-time interactive 3D tumor segmentation using a fast level-set algorithm. J Med Imaging Health Inf 5(8):1998–2002. doi:10.1166/jmihi.2015.1685
24. Whitaker RT (1998) A level-set approach to 3D reconstruction from range data. Int J Comput Vis 29(3):203–231. doi:10.1023/A:1008036829907
25. Zheng Y, Barbu A, Georgescu B, Scheuering M, Comaniciu D (2008) Four-chamber heart modeling and automatic segmentation for 3-D cardiac CT volumes using marginal space learning and steerable features. IEEE Trans Med Imaging 27(11):1668–1681. doi:10.1109/TMI.2008.2004421

Chapter 11
Automatic Multiorgan Segmentation Using Hierarchically Registered Probabilistic Atlases

Razmig Kéchichian, Sébastien Valette and Michel Desvignes

Abstract We propose a generic method for the automatic multiple-organ segmentation of 3D images based on a multilabel graph cut optimization approach which uses location likelihood of organs and prior information of spatial relationships between them. The latter is derived from shortest-path constraints defined on the adjacency graph of structures and the former is defined by probabilistic atlases learned from a training dataset. Organ atlases are mapped to the image by a fast (2+1)D hierarchical registration method based on SURF keypoints. Registered atlases are also used to derive organ intensity likelihoods. Prior and likelihood models are then introduced in a joint centroidal Voronoi image clustering and graph cut multiobject segmentation framework. Qualitative and quantitative evaluation has been performed on contrast-enhanced CT and MR images from the VISCERAL dataset.

11.1 Introduction and Related Work

Clinical practice today, especially whole-body CT and MR imaging, often generates large numbers of high-resolution images, which makes tasks of efficient data access, transfer, analysis and visualization challenging. This is especially true in distributed

R. Kéchichian (✉) · S. Valette
CREATIS, CNRS UMR5220, Inserm U1044, INSA-Lyon,
Université de Lyon, Lyon, France
e-mail: razmig.kechichian@creatis.insa-lyon.fr

S. Valette
e-mail: sebastien.valette@creatis.insa-lyon.fr

R. Kéchichian · S. Valette
Université Claude Bernard Lyon 1, Lyon, France

M. Desvignes
GIPSA-Lab, CNRS UMR 5216, Grenoble-INP, Université Joseph Fourier,
Saint Martin d'Héres, France
e-mail: michel.desvignes@gipsa-lab.grenoble-inp.fr

M. Desvignes
Université Stendhal, Saint Martin d'Héres, France

© The Author(s) 2017
A. Hanbury et al. (eds.), *Cloud-Based Benchmarking
of Medical Image Analysis*, DOI 10.1007/978-3-319-49644-3_11

computing environments which have seen a growing use of hand-held terminals for interactive data access and visualization of anatomy. Therefore, there is great interest in efficient and robust medical image segmentation algorithms for the purposes of creating patient-specific anatomical models, clinical applications, medical research and education, and visualization and semantic navigation of full-body anatomy [3, 26].

Traditionally, single-object- or pathology-oriented, recent image processing methods [9, 12, 14, 15, 19, 23, 25, 27] have made the analysis and the segmentation of multiple anatomical structures increasingly possible. However, CT and MR images have intrinsic characteristics that render their automatic segmentation challenging. They are commonly degraded by various noise sources and artefacts due to limited acquisition time and resolution, and patient motion which all reduce the prominence of intensity edges in images. In addition, MR images suffer from spatial distortion of tissue intensity due to main magnetic field inhomogeneity. Regardless of the imaging modality and related artefacts, many anatomically and functionally distinct structures, especially those corresponding to soft tissues, have similar intensity levels in images and, furthermore, blend into surrounding tissues which have intensities close to their own. It is impossible to identify and segment such structures automatically on the basis of intensity information only. Hence, most advanced segmentation methods exploit some form of prior information on structure location [12, 19, 27] or interrelations [9, 14, 23, 25] to achieve greater robustness and precision. Hierarchical approaches to segmentation [23, 25, 32] rely on hierarchical organizations of prior information and algorithms that proceed in a coarse-to-fine manner according to anatomical level of detail.

Graph cut methods, which have been widely applied to single-object segmentation problems [4], rely on a maximum-flow binary optimization scheme of a discrete cost function on the image graph. For a particular class of cost functions which frequently arises in segmentation applications [16], these methods produce provably good approximate solutions in multiobject [5] and global optima in single-object segmentation. In addition, simultaneous multiobject segmentation approaches are superior to their sequential counterparts in that they raise questions neither on the best segmentation sequence to follow nor on how to avoid the propagation of errors of individual segmentations [9].

While widely used by the computer vision community, keypoint-based image description and matching methods, such as SIFT [20] and SURF [2], have found relatively few application proposals in medical image processing. These methods proceed by first detecting some points of interest (edges, ridges, blobs, etc.) within the image, then compute vectors describing local neighbourhoods around these points and use them as content descriptors. The approach has been successfully applied to image indexing, content-based image retrieval, object detection and recognition, and image registration [30]. In medical imaging, 3D versions of SIFT have been used in brain MR image matching [6], linear registration of radiation therapy data [1], and nonlinear (deformable) registration of thoracic CT [31] and brain MR [22] images. A SURF-based method [10] has also been successfully applied to the intermodality registration of 2D brain images. A review of keypoint-based medical image registration can be found in [28].

We propose a generic method for the automatic multiple-organ segmentation of 3D images based on multilabel graph cut optimization which uses location and intensity likelihoods of organs and prior information of their spatial configuration. The spatial prior is derived from shortest-path pairwise constraints defined on the adjacency graph of structures [14], and the organ location likelihood is defined by probabilistic atlases [24] learned from the VISCERAL training dataset [11]. We register organ atlases to the image prior to segmentation using a fast (2+1)D registration method based on SURF keypoints. Registered atlases are also used to derive organ intensity likelihoods. Prior and likelihood models are then introduced in a joint centroidal Voronoi image clustering and graph cut multiobject segmentation framework. We present the results of qualitative and quantitative evaluation of our method on contrast-enhanced CT and MR images from the VISCERAL dataset.

11.2   Methods

In the following, we present the different elements of our approach in detail, namely the keypoint-based image registration method and its use in organ atlas construction as well as its hierarchical application in segmentation. Image clustering and segmentation methods are detailed next, followed by a presentation of evaluation results in the subsequent section.

11.2.1   SURF Keypoint-Based Image Registration

We first outline our fast (2+1)D algorithm for the rigid registration of 3D medical images using content features. Our method has the following properties:

- Features are extracted in 2D volume slices. This has the advantage of being fast and easily parallelizable. Another advantage is that medical data are usually stored in a picture archiving and communication system (PACS) in the form of volume slices as opposed to full 3D volumes. Our method easily fits into such medical environments. Note that while feature extraction is done in 2D images, registration is still performed in 3D, hence the (2+1)D definition.
- Partial matching is well handled, thus making our algorithm suitable for general medical data.
- Total processing time is on the order of seconds.
- The (2+1)D paradigm currently restricts our method to image volumes with consistent orientations. A pair of images featuring patients with orthogonal orientations cannot be registered for now.

11.2.1.1   2D Feature Extraction and Matching

As previously mentioned, we extract features from 2D slices of the image volume. We currently use the SURF image descriptor [21]; however, our method is generic and would work with other descriptors as well. To reduce computation time, we first downsample the input volume to a user-specified size. As a rule of thumb, we isotropically resample each volume so that its second longest dimension is equal to the desired resolution R. For example, with $R = 100$, the VISCERAL training dataset image 10000108_1_CTce_ThAb of dimensions $512 \times 512 \times 468$ and spacing $0.7\,\text{mm} \times 0.7\,\text{mm} \times 1.5\,\text{mm}$ is resampled to a $100 \times 100 \times 198$ volume with an isotropic spacing of $3.54\,\text{mm}$.

Next, we extract 2D SURF features from each slice. As these operations are completely independent, this step is carried out in a parallel manner. Figure 11.1 shows feature extraction results on a pair of axial slices from VISCERAL training dataset images 10000108_1_CTce_ThAb (left) and 10000109_1_CTce_ThAb (right). The top row shows all features extracted from these slices. The number of extracted features is 11500 and 9400, respectively.

Once all features are extracted, they are matched using the widely used second closest ratio criterion [20]. If the first volume V_1 contains n_1 slices and the second volume V_2 contains n_2 slices, we have to compute $n_1 \times n_2$ image matches, which again is easily carried out in a parallel fashion. The bottom row of Fig. 11.1 shows the nine matching couples (pairs of keypoints) found in both slices.

The output of the matching step is a similarity matrix S of $n_1 \times n_2$ of, possibly empty, matching couple sets $H_{i,j}$. Figure 11.2 illustrates the 2D matching procedure on test images 10000108_1_CTce_ThAb and 10000109_1_CTce_ThAb. Figure 11.3 shows similarity matrices reflecting the number of matching couples between any pair of slices for three settings of downsampling resolution R (grey level is inversely proportional to the number of matching couples). Matrix diagonals are clearly visible, confirming the fact that input volumes contain similar structures. In total, 2561 matching couples were found between this pair of volumes with $R = 100$.

11.2.1.2   (2+1)D Registration

Once 2D matches are found, we are able to proceed with volume registration. For robustness purposes, we use a simple "scale + translation" transformation model:

$$\begin{bmatrix} x' \\ y' \\ z' \end{bmatrix} = s \begin{bmatrix} x \\ y \\ z \end{bmatrix} + \begin{bmatrix} t_x \\ t_y \\ t_z \end{bmatrix} . \tag{11.1}$$

We estimate the four parameters s, t_x, t_y and t_z in similar spirit to the RANSAC method [8], using the set of matching couples between the slices of the pair of volumes, computed as indicated in the previous subsection. RANSAC is an iterative

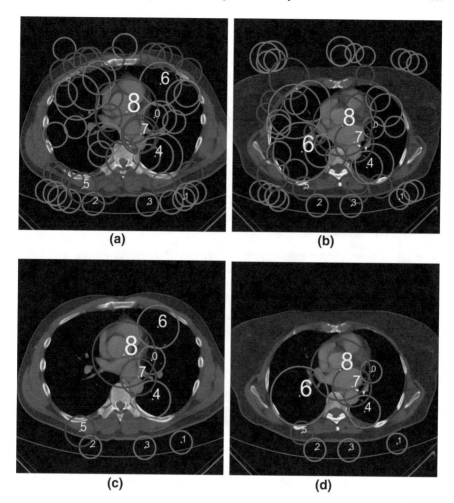

Fig. 11.1 Matching two slices of images. **a** `10000108_1_CTce_ThAb` and **b** `10000109_1_CTce_ThAb` from the VISCERAL training dataset. **a, b** Show all features found in both slices (a feature is represented by a *circle*). **c, d** Show the nine matching features between the two slices. *Blue* and *red circles* correspond to positive and negative Laplacian values [2]

parametric model estimation method known to be very efficient in the presence of outliers. One RANSAC iteration usually consists in randomly picking a small number of samples to estimate the model parameters, then counting the number of data samples consistent with the model, rejecting outliers. After performing all iterations, the model providing the highest number of consistent data samples is kept as the solution. In our case, we carry out parameter estimation in a two-stage fashion; first, we fix the parameters s and t_z which allow us to work only on a subset of S, then we estimate the remaining parameters t_x and t_y. More specifically, we carry out the nth RANSAC iteration as follows:

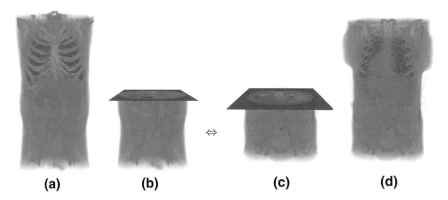

(a)   **(b)**   **(c)**   **(d)**

Fig. 11.2 Feature matching. The two input volumes (**a**, **b**) are sliced (**c**, **d**), and each slice from the first volume is compared against every slice from the second volume

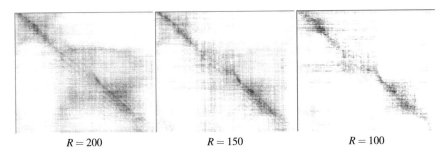

$R = 200$ $R = 150$ $R = 100$

Fig. 11.3 Similarity matrices of test volumes `10000108_1_CTce_ThAb` and `10000109_1_CTce_ThAb` for different values of downsampling resolution R

- Randomly pick a line L_n crossing S. This fixes half of the transform parameters, that is, the parameters s and t_z. The top row of Fig. 11.4 shows three different randomly picked lines on S.
- Build the couple set M_n as the union of all couple sets $H_{i,j}$ in S within a distance d_L to L_n. In our experiments, we set d_L to 2.5. For the three cases illustrated in the top row of Fig. 11.4, couple sets M_n correspond to image pixels covered by the red lines.
- Randomly pick one couple from M_n, which allows to estimate the remaining transform parameters t_x and t_y.
- Count the number of couples N_n in M_n which are consistent with the transform, excluding outliers and forbidding any keypoints to appear in multiple matching couples. If f_1 and f_2 are the coordinates of a couple, consistency checking is done by transforming the coordinates of f_1 into f_1' using Eq. 11.1, and verifying that f_1' is within a fixed distance d_c from f_2. In practice, we set d_c to 20 mm.

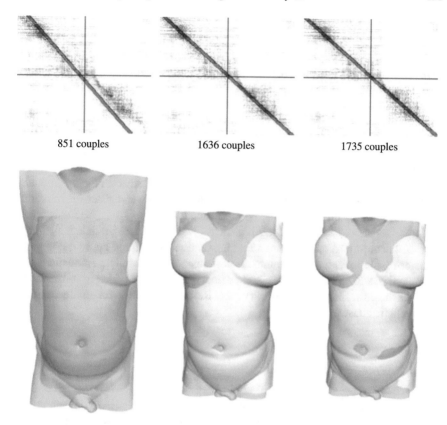

851 couples   1636 couples   1735 couples

Fig. 11.4 (2+1)D registration of test volumes `10000108_1_CTce_ThAb` and `10000109_1_CTce_ThAb`. The *top row* shows three randomly picked lines L_n on the similarity matrix and their respective numbers of matching couples. The *bottom row* shows the corresponding registrations of test volumes, showing only patient body envelopes

In all experiments, we perform 2×10^5 iterations to register a pair of volumes. The bottom row of Fig. 11.4 illustrates the final registration of test images `10000108_1_CTce_ThAb` and `10000109_1_CTce_ThAb` showing only respective patient body envelopes.

11.2.2 Organ Atlas Construction

Using contrast-enhanced CT and MR images and available ground-truth annotations from the VISCERAL training dataset, we construct modality-specific probabilistic atlases for the following 20 structures: thyroid; trachea; sternum; liver; spleen; pancreas; gall bladder; first lumbar vertebra; aorta; urinary bladder; right and left lungs, kidneys, adrenal glands, psoas major and rectus abdominis muscle bodies. In addition, we create atlases for three additional image and body regions: background (BKG), thorax and abdomen (THAB) and a body envelope (ENV) from annotations generated automatically as follows. BKG is created by thresholding the image followed by morphological processing in order to isolate the background from the body region. THAB is created as the dilated union of the aforementioned 20 structures and their bounding 3D ellipse, from which the structures are subtracted after dilation. Finally, ENV is defined as the image minus BKG and THAB. Note that ENV is a crude body envelope that comprises skin, fat, muscle and bone structures. Figure 11.8c, f illustrate the additional annotations.

To create probabilistic atlases, we choose a representative image per modality from the dataset and use it as a reference onto which we register all remaining images in the modality via the method described in Sect. 11.2.1. We register each structure separately in a bounding box of a given margin in the intensity image, defined according to the corresponding annotation image, and apply the obtained transform subsequently to the annotation image. We accumulate annotations thus registered in a 3D histogram of reference image dimensions which is normalized to produce the corresponding probability map. Refer to Fig. 11.6a for an illustration of probabilistic atlases.

11.2.3 Image Clustering

The full-resolution voxel representation is often redundant because objects usually comprise many similar voxels that could be grouped. Therefore, we simplify the image prior to segmentation by an image-adaptive centroidal Voronoi tessellation (CVT), which strikes a good balance between cluster compactness and object boundary adherence and helps to place subsequent segmentation boundaries precisely. We have shown that the clustering step improves the overall run-time and memory footprint of the segmentation process up to an order of magnitude without compromising the quality of the result [14].

Let us define a greyscale image as a set of voxels $\mathscr{I} = \{v \mid v = (x, y, z)\}$ and associate with each voxel $v \in \mathscr{I}$ a grey level I_v from some range $I \subset \mathbb{R}$. Given a greyscale image $\mathscr{I}$ and n sites $c_i \in \mathscr{I}$, a CVT partitions $\mathscr{I}$ into n disjoint clusters C_i associated with each centroid c_i and minimizes the following energy:

$$F(v; c_i) = \sum_{i=1}^{n} \left(\sum_{v \in C_i} \rho(v) \left(\|v - c_i\|^2 + \alpha \|I_v - I_i\|^2 \right) \right). \qquad (11.2)$$

In Eq. 11.2, $\rho(v)$ is a density function defined according to the intensity gradient magnitude at voxel v, $\rho(v) = |\nabla I_v|$, α is a positive scalar and I_i is the grey level of the cluster C_i defined as the mean intensity of its voxels. Intuitively, minimizing Eq. 11.2 corresponds to maximizing cluster compactness in terms of both geometry

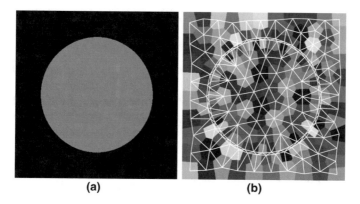

(a)   **(b)**

Fig. 11.5 An image-adaptive CVT clustering and its dual graph for a circle image

and grey level. Refer to Fig. 11.5 for an illustration in 2D. To minimize Eq. 11.2, we apply a variant of the clustering algorithm in [7], which approximates a CVT in a computationally efficient manner, involving only local queries on voxels located on boundaries of pairs of clusters.

For referral in later sections, we shall define the graph of a CVT, illustrated in Fig. 11.5b. Denote the surface of a cluster C_i by ∂C_i. Given a CVT clustering $\mathscr{C}$, let the set $\mathscr{S}$ index its clusters, and let $\mathscr{G} = \langle \mathscr{S}, \mathscr{E} \rangle$ be an undirected graph on cluster centroids where pairs of clusters having nonzero area common surface define the set of edges $\mathscr{E} = \{\{i, j\} \mid i, j \in \mathscr{S}, |\partial C_i \cap \partial C_j| \neq 0\}$. Consequently, the neighbourhood of a node $i \in \mathscr{S}$ is defined as $\mathscr{N}_i = \{j \mid j \in \mathscr{S}, \exists \{i, j\} \in \mathscr{E}\}$.

11.2.4 Multiorgan Image Segmentation

We formulate image segmentation as a labelling problem, defined as the assignment of a label from a set of labels L representing the structures to be segmented to each of the variables in a set of n variables, indexed by $\mathscr{S}$, corresponding to the clusters of a CVT-clustered image. Assume that each variable $i \in \mathscr{S}$ is associated with the corresponding node in the graph $\mathscr{G}$ of the CVT defined in Sect. 11.2.3. An assignment of labels to all variables is called a configuration and is denoted by $\ell \in \mathscr{L}$. An assignment of a label to a single variable is denoted by ℓ_i. We cast the labelling problem in a maximum a posteriori estimation framework and solve it by minimizing the following energy function of label configurations via the expansion moves multilabel graph cut algorithm [5], which has been shown to outperform popular multilabel optimization algorithms in terms of both speed and quality of obtained solutions [29]:

$$E(\ell) = t_1 \sum_{i \in \mathscr{S}} D_i(\ell_i) + t_2 \sum_{i \in \mathscr{S}} P_i(\ell_i) + \frac{1}{2} \sum_{i \in \mathscr{S}} \sum_{j \in \mathscr{N}_i} V_{i,j}(\ell_i, \ell_j) \ . \qquad (11.3)$$

In Eq. 11.3, t_1 and t_2 are temperature hyperparameters, and $\mathscr{N}_i$ is the neighbourhood of the variable $i \in \mathscr{S}$. The first and second sums in Eq. 11.3 correspond, respectively, to organ intensity and location (atlas) likelihood energies, and the third is the energy of a prior distribution of label configurations expressed as a Markov random field [18] with respect to the graph $\mathscr{G}$. We shall define these terms in detail.

11.2.4.1 Spatial Configuration Prior

Pairwise terms of Eq. 11.3 encode prior information on interactions between labels assigned to pairs of neighbouring variables encouraging the spatial consistency of labelling with respect to a reference model. We define these terms according to the piecewise-constant vicinity prior model proposed in [14], which, unlike the standard Potts model, incurs multiple levels of penalization capturing the spatial configuration of structures in multiobject segmentation. It is defined as follows. Let $\mathscr{R}$ be the set of symmetric adjacency relations on pairs of distinct labels (corresponding to image structures), $\mathscr{R} = \{r \mid a\,r\,b, \ a, b \in L, \ a \neq b\}$. $\mathscr{R}$ can be represented by a weighted undirected graph on L, $\mathscr{A} = \langle L, W \rangle$, with the set of edges $W = \big\{ \{a, b\} \mid \exists r \in \mathscr{R}, \ a\,r\,b, \ a \neq b \big\}$, where edge weights are defined by $w(\{a, b\}) = 1$, such that $w(\{a, b\}) = \infty$ if $\nexists r \in \mathscr{R}, \ a\,r\,b$.

Given the graph $\mathscr{A}$, we define the pairwise term in Eq. 11.3 as follows:

$$V_{i,j}(\ell_i, \ell_j) = |\partial C_i \cap \partial C_j|\,\omega(a, b), \quad \ell_i = a, \ \ell_j = b \ . \qquad (11.4)$$

where $\omega(a, b)$ is the shortest-path weight from a to b in $\mathscr{A}$. The adjacency graph of structures according to which we define the spatial prior in our experiments is given in Fig. 11.6b. In Eq. 11.4, the area of the common surface of adjacent clusters $|\partial C_i \cap \partial C_j|$ is introduced, so that $\forall a, b \in L$ the sum of pairwise energies in (11.3) is equal to the area of the common surface between the corresponding pair of structures multiplied by the shortest-path weight. This definition ensures that the segmentation energy is independent of the CVT clustering resolution [13].

11.2.4.2 Intensity and Location Likelihoods

Unary terms of Eq. 11.3 measure the cost of assigning labels to variables. They are defined as negative log-likelihood functions derived from organ observed intensity and location probabilities:

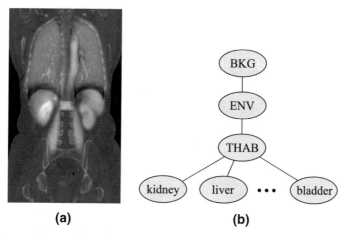

Fig. 11.6 **a** Registered organ atlases overlaid on a CT image and **b** the adjacency graph used to define the spatial prior

$$D_i(\ell_i) = -\ln \prod_{v \in C_i} \Pr(I_v \mid \ell_i) , \tag{11.5a}$$

$$P_i(\ell_i) = -\ln \prod_{v \in C_i} \Pr(X_v \mid \ell_i) . \tag{11.5b}$$

In Eq. 11.5b, X_v denotes the object-space coordinates of the voxel v. Conditional probabilities in Eq. 11.5a and 11.5b correspond, respectively, to those of voxel intensity and location given the structure ℓ_i. To estimate the conditional probability distribution $\Pr(I \mid l)$ for a given label $l \in L$, we first register the corresponding organ atlas to the image, then estimate the conditional probability as a Gauss-smoothed and normalized intensity histogram derived from voxels in high-probability regions of the registered atlas according to a threshold value. Conditional probability distributions $\Pr(X \mid L)$ are defined directly from registered atlases. The next section outlines our hierarchical registration method which maps organ atlases to an image prior to its segmentation.

11.2.4.3 Hierarchical Registration of Organ Atlases

We register probabilistic organ atlases, constructed as described in Sect. 11.2.2, to an image in a three-step hierarchical fashion starting at the full image scale, then on an intermediate level corresponding to the THAB region and finally on individual organs. After performing registration on each scale, we apply the obtained transform to the corresponding atlas as well as to those of organs contained in the registered region. As in Sect. 11.2.2, we register each structure separately in a bounding box of a given margin in the intensity image, defined according to the corresponding atlas.

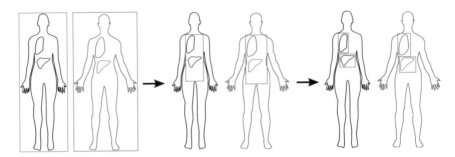

Fig. 11.7 An illustration of the proposed hierarchical registration procedure

Figure 11.7 illustrates the hierarchical registration procedure, and Fig. 11.6a gives an example of registered organ atlases overlaid on the CT image to which they have been registered.

11.3 Evaluation Results and Discussion

We have carried out qualitative evaluation on several contrast-enhanced CT and MR images from the VISCERAL training dataset. Figure 11.8 shows a pair of segmentations on images `10000109_1_CTce_ThAb` and `10000324_4_MRT1cefs_Ab`. Their dimensions, respectively, are $512 \times 512 \times 428$ and $312 \times 72 \times 384$. For this pair of images, the number of CVT clusters is set, respectively, to 3 and 20% of image voxel count. In all experiments, we set temperature parameters t_1 and t_2 so that intensity and location likelihood-based unary terms have the same magnitude in Eq. 11.3. Likewise, for intensity likelihood estimation in all experiments, we fix the probability threshold mentioned in Sect. 11.2.4.2 to 0.9 times that of the maximum probability of the registered probabilistic atlas. The spatial configuration prior is defined according to the adjacency graph given in Fig. 11.6b. We note that, due to a smaller field of view, VISCERAL dataset contrast-enhanced MR images exclude thoracic organs, namely the pair of lungs, the trachea, the sternum and the thyroid. Naturally, we do not construct probabilistic atlases for these structures nor do we take them into account for the segmentation of MR images.

Table 11.1 presents the results of quantitative evaluation of our segmentation method on contrast-enhanced CT images during the VISCERAL Anatomy 2 Benchmark and those of its more recent evaluation on contrast-enhanced MR images. We report results corresponding to the best setting of temperature parameters out of the allowed five. For CT images, the settings for t_1 are as follows: 0.15, 0.20, 0.25, 0.30 and 0.40. For MR images, tested settings of this parameter are as follows: 0.6, 0.8, 1.0, 1.2 and 1.4. The parameter t_2 was set to $0.2\,t_1$ in both cases. These ranges of parameter values were experimentally found to give the best results in offline evaluations on the VISCERAL training dataset. For each structure, the Table 11.1 gives the

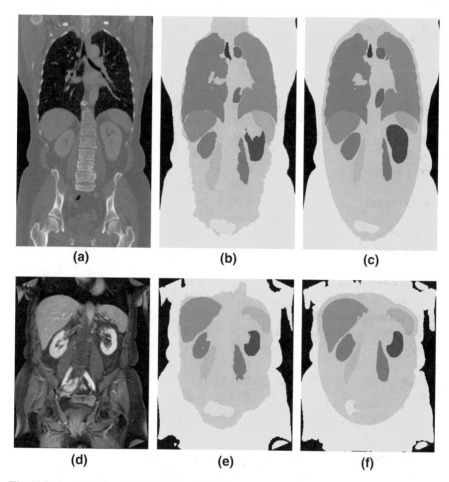

Fig. 11.8 Segmentation of VISCERAL training dataset images `10000109_1_CTce_ThAb` (top row) and `10000324_4_MRT1cefs_Ab` (*bottom row*). Coronal sections correspond to **a, d** the image, **b, e** its segmentation and **c, f** the associated ground truth with additional labels for BKG, ENV and THAB regions

number of produced segmentations out of an attempted 10, mean Dice and average distance (in millimeters) measurements. "N/A" indicates an absent structure, while a dash "–" indicates one for which the segmentation was missed or was not attempted.

Mean run-time and memory footprint figures of our algorithm are given in Table 11.2. These measurements are taken on the 20 contrast-enhanced CT images in the VISCERAL training dataset, the average dimension of which is $512 \times 512 \times 426$. The number of CVT clusters is set to 5% of image voxel count. The algorithm is run on a cluster computer of heterogeneous nodes with an average CPU speed of 2.1 GHz, an average number of cores of 20 and an average memory size of 87 GB.

Table 11.1 Quantitative evaluation results of the proposed method on contrast-enhanced CT and MR images

Structures	CT			MR		
	#	Dice	Avg. Dist.	#	Dice	Avg. Dist.
Trachea	9	0.62	18.56	N/A	N/A	N/A
Lung (R)	10	0.95	0.30	N/A	N/A	N/A
Lung (L)	10	0.96	0.20	N/A	N/A	N/A
Pancreas	7	0.35	11.45	6	0.37	11.99
Gall bladder	2	0.14	21.82	1	0.30	1.90
Urinary bladder	10	0.77	1.08	10	0.40	3.67
Sternum	10	0.63	6.59	N/A	N/A	N/A
Lumbar vertebra	10	0.49	9.74	7	0.26	6.65
Kidney (R)	10	0.81	1.81	10	0.80	3.90
Kidney (L)	10	0.86	0.89	8	0.74	1.69
Adrenal gland (R)	–	–	–	–	–	–
Adrenal gland (L)	–	–	–	–	–	–
Psoas major muscle (R)	10	0.71	2.70	10	0.69	1.73
Psoas major muscle (L)	10	0.79	1.22	10	0.66	2.28
Rectus abdominis muscle (R)	9	0.26	30.25	–	–	–
Rectus abdominis muscle (L)	10	0.13	24.43	–	–	–
Aorta	10	0.58	5.43	3	0.27	17.40
Liver	10	0.93	0.34	10	0.77	1.91
Thyroid	3	0.04	13.77	N/A	N/A	N/A
Spleen	10	0.84	1.29	9	0.53	3.31

Table 11.2 Mean memory footprint and run-time figures of proposed algorithms measured on 20 contrast-enhanced CT images from the VISCERAL training dataset

Memory (MB)	Registration (s)	Clustering (s)	Segmentation (s)	Total run-time (m)
10520.87	4294.60	8995.20	2598.48	264.80

From these results, we can readily see that our method performs better on CT than on MR images. This is due to the fact that tissues in CT images have consistent appearances, whereas in MR images, they suffer intensity inhomogeneity. In addition, MR images in the VISCERAL dataset have lower resolution compared to CT images. We can observe furthermore that our method performs better on larger, well-contrasted structures than on smaller, low-contrasted ones such as the gall bladder, the thyroid and the adrenal glands. This is mainly due to the inaccurate localization of these structures by our registration method and the subsequent flawed estimation of the structure intensity likelihood. For most structures however, even though our hierarchical approach of mapping atlases to the image relies on a rigid registration method, unlike many hierarchical methods which use non-rigid deformable registration [17], it helps localizing structure boundaries in segmentation quite well. This is because location information roughly registered atlases provide is complemented by intensity similarity and spatial consistency criteria. Furthermore, full-body modelling by the introduction of BKG, ENV and THAB annotations not only complements location information and allows for hierarchical registration, but also increases the discriminative power of the spatial prior by a higher penalization of inconsistent configurations.

11.4 Concluding Remarks and Future Work

It should not go without notice that without the VISCERAL platform and the dataset, we would not have been able to test and understand the limits and the properties of our algorithms, to improve them and to develop new ones. We hope that our active participation in benchmarks and our regular feedback on software and data have been valuable for the VISCERAL project.

We are currently scrutinizing our hierarchical registration method in view of multiresolution extensions, possibly bypassing anatomical hierarchy, which would help better localize structures, especially small, low-contrasted ones. We are also investigating the introduction of a better, more robust intensity likelihood estimation method. If an inaccurate registration could be detected and quantified, then it may be possible to "correct" it. Otherwise, with a large training dataset to draw upon, techniques from machine learning could easily be used. Another interesting venue for future research is the extension of the spatial prior model to express other types of relations, such as spatial directionality, and the possibility of taking into account the uncertainty of relations.

References

1. Allaire S, Kim JJ, Breen SL, Jaffray DA, Pekar V (2008) Full orientation invariance and improved feature selectivity of 3D SIFT with application to medical image analysis. In: IEEE CVPRW, pp 1–8
2. Bay H, Ess A, Tuytelaars T, Van Gool L (2008) Speeded-up robust features (SURF). Comput Vis Image Underst 110(3):346–359
3. Blume A, Chun W, Kogan D, Kokkevis V, Weber N, Petterson RW, Zeiger R (2011) Google body: 3D human anatomy in the browser. In: ACM SIGGRAPH 2011 Talks, p 19:1
4. Boykov Y, Funka-Lea G (2006) Graph cuts and efficient N-D image segmentation. Int J Comput Vis 70(2):109–131
5. Boykov Y, Veksler O, Zabih R (2001) Fast approximate energy minimization via graph cuts. IEEE Trans Pattern Anal Mach Intell 23(11):1222–1239
6. Cheung W, Hamarneh G (2009) n-SIFT: n-dimensional scale invariant feature transform. IEEE Trans Image Process 18(9):2012–2021
7. Dardenne J, Valette S, Siauve N, Burais N, Prost R (2009) Variational tetraedral mesh generation from discrete volume data. Vis Comput 25(5):401–410

8. Fischler MA, Bolles RC (1981) Random sample consensus: a paradigm for model fitting with applications to image analysis and automated cartography. Commun ACM 24(6):381–395

9. Fouquier G, Atif J, Bloch I (2012) Sequential model-based segmentation and recognition of image structures driven by visual features and spatial relations. Comput Vis Image Underst 116(1):146–165

10. Gu Z, Cai L, Yin Y, Ding Y, Kan H (2014) Registration of brain medical images based on SURF algorithm and RANSAC algorithm. TELKOMNIKA Indones J Electr Eng 12(3):2290–2297

11. Hanbury A, Müller H, Langs G, Weber MA, Menze BH, Fernandez TS (2012) Bringing the algorithms to the data: cloud–based benchmarking for medical image analysis. In: Catarci T, Forner P, Hiemstra D, Peñas A, Santucci G (eds) CLEF 2012. LNCS, vol 7488. Springer, Heidelberg, pp 24–29. doi:10.1007/978-3-642-33247-0_3

12. Iglesias JE, Konukoglu E, Montillo A, Tu Z, Criminisi A (2011) Combining generative and discriminative models for semantic segmentation of CT scans via active learning. In: Székely G, Hahn HK (eds) IPMI 2011. LNCS, vol 6801. Springer, Heidelberg, pp 25–36. doi:10.1007/978-3-642-22092-0_3

13. Kéchichian R (2013) Structural priors for multiobject semiautomatic segmentation of three-dimensional medical images via clustering and graph cut algorithms. PhD thesis, Université de Lyon

14. Kéchichian R, Valette S, Desvignes M, Prost R (2013) Shortest-path constraints for 3D multi-object semi-automatic segmentation via clustering and graph cut. IEEE Trans Image Process 22(11):4224–4236

15. Kohlberger T, Sofka M, Zhang J, Birkbeck N, Wetzl J, Kaftan J, Declerck J, Zhou SK (2011) Automatic multi-organ segmentation using learning-based segmentation and level set optimization. In: Fichtinger G, Martel A, Peters T (eds) MICCAI 2011. LNCS, vol 6893. Springer, Heidelberg, pp 338–345. doi:10.1007/978-3-642-23626-6_42

16. Kolmogorov V, Zabih R (2004) What energy functions can be minimized via graph cuts? IEEE Trans Pattern Anal Mach Intell 26(2):147–159

17. Lester H, Arridge SR (1999) A survey of hierarchical non-linear medical image registration. Pattern Recognit 32(1):129–149

18. Li SZ (2009) Markov random field modeling in image analysis. Springer, Berlin

19. Linguraru MG, Pura JA, Pamulapati V, Summers RM (2012) Statistical 4D graphs for multi-organ abdominal segmentation from multiphase CT. Med Image Anal 16(4):904–914

20. Lowe DG (2004) Distinctive image features from scale-invariant keypoints. Int J Comput Vis 60(2):91–110

21. Lukashevich P, Zalesky B, Ablameyko S (2011) Medical image registration based on SURF detector. Pattern Recognit Image Anal 21(3):519–521

22. Moradi M, Abolmaesoumi P, Mousavi P (2006) Deformable registration using scale space keypoints. In: Medical imaging, international society for optics and photonics, p 61442G

23. Okada T, Linguraru MG, Yoshida Y, Hori M, Summers RM, Chen Y-W, Tomiyama N, Sato Y (2012) Abdominal multi-organ segmentation of CT images based on hierarchical spatial modeling of organ interrelations. In: Yoshida H, Sakas G, Linguraru MG (eds) ABD-MICCAI 2011. LNCS, vol 7029. Springer, Heidelberg, pp 173–180. doi:10.1007/978-3-642-28557-8_22

24. Park H, Bland PH, Meyer CR (2003) Construction of an abdominal probabilistic atlas and its application in segmentation. IEEE Trans Med Imag 22(4):483–492

25. Seifert S, Barbu A, Zhou SK, Liu D, Feulner J, Huber M, Suehling M, Cavallaro A, Comaniciu D (2009) Hierarchical parsing and semantic navigation of full body CT data. In: SPIE Medical Imaging, Lake Buena Vista, FL, USA

26. Seifert S, Kelm M, Moeller M, Mukherjee S, Cavallaro A, Huber M, Comaniciu D (2010) Semantic annotation of medical images. In: SPIE medical imaging, international society for optics and photonics, p 762, 808

27. Song Z, Tustison N, Avants B, Gee J (2006) Adaptive graph cuts with tissue priors for brain MRI segmentation. In: IEEE ISBI, pp 762–765

28. Sotiras A, Davatzikos C, Paragios N (2013) Deformable medical image registration: a survey. IEEE Trans Med Imag 32(7):1153–1190
29. Szeliski R, Zabih R, Scharstein D, Veksler O, Kolmogorov V, Agarwala A, Tappen M, Rother C (2008) A comparative study of energy minimization methods for markov random fields with smoothness-based priors. IEEE Trans Pattern Anal Mach Intell 30(6):1068–1080
30. Tuytelaars T, Mikolajczyk K (2008) Local invariant feature detectors: a survey. Found Trends Comput Gr Vis 3(3):177–280
31. Urschler M, Bauer J, Ditt H, Bischof H (2006) SIFT and shape context for feature-based nonlinear registration of thoracic CT images. In: Beichel RR, Sonka M (eds) CVAMIA 2006. LNCS, vol 4241. Springer, Heidelberg, pp 73–84. doi:10.1007/11889762_7
32. Wolz R, Chu C, Misawa K, Mori K, Rueckert D (2012) Multi-organ abdominal CT segmentation using hierarchically weighted subject-specific atlases. In: Ayache N, Delingette H, Golland P, Mori K (eds) MICCAI 2012. LNCS, vol 7510. Springer, Heidelberg, pp 10–17. doi:10.1007/978-3-642-33415-3_2

Chapter 12
Multiatlas Segmentation Using Robust Feature-Based Registration

**Frida Fejne, Matilda Landgren, Jennifer Alvén, Johannes Ulén,
Johan Fredriksson, Viktor Larsson, Olof Enqvist and Fredrik Kahl**

Abstract This paper presents a pipeline which uses a multiatlas approach for multiorgan segmentation in whole-body CT images. In order to obtain accurate registrations between the target and the atlas images, we develop an adapted feature-based method which uses organ-specific features. These features are learnt during an offline preprocessing step, and thus, the algorithm still benefits from the speed of feature-based registration methods. These feature sets are then used to obtain pairwise non-rigid transformations using RANSAC followed by a thin-plate spline refinement or NIFTYREG. The fusion of the transferred atlas labels is performed using a random forest classifier, and finally, the segmentation is obtained using graph cuts with a Potts model as interaction term. Our pipeline was evaluated on 20 organs in 10 whole-body CT images at the VISCERAL Anatomy Challenge, in conjunction

---

F. Fejne and M. Landgren—The authors assert equal contribution and joint first authorship.

F. Fejne · J. Alvén · O. Enqvist · F. Kahl
Department of Signals and Systems, Chalmers University of Technology,
Gothenburg, Sweden
e-mail: fejne@chalmers.se

J. Alvén
e-mail: alven@chalmers.se

O. Enqvist
e-mail: olof.enqvist@chalmers.se

F. Kahl
e-mail: fredrik.kahl@chalmers.se

M. Landgren (✉) · J. Ulén · J. Fredriksson · V. Larsson · F. Kahl
Centre for Mathematical Sciences, Lund University, Lund, Sweden
e-mail: matilda@maths.lth.se

J. Ulén
e-mail: ulen@maths.lth.se

J. Fredriksson
e-mail: johanf@maths.lth.se

V. Larsson
e-mail: viktorl@maths.lth.se

with the International Symposium on Biomedical Imaging, Brooklyn, New York, in April 2015. It performed best on majority of the organs, with respect to the Dice index.

12.1 Introduction

Segmentation of anatomical structures is a fundamental task in medical image analysis. It has several applications such as localization of organs, detection of tumours or other pathological structures, and the results can, for example, serve as input to computer-aided diagnosis (CAD) systems. Multiorgan segmentation is useful, e.g. in radiotherapy planning [25], where not only the location of the tumour is of most interest, but also the location of the surrounding (vital) organs. Furthermore, it can also be used in the preparation of and during computer-assisted surgery [30]. Automated methods are preferable due to the time-consuming task to do the segmentations manually and the need of a skilled expert.

In this paper, we propose a pipeline that uses a multiatlas approach for an automatic multiorgan segmentation for CT images. The segmentation of each organ is independent of the others and we show that very reliable organ localization can be obtained using (i) robust optimization techniques for registration, (ii) learned feature correspondences and (iii) refinement with a random forest classifier and graph cut segmentation.

12.1.1 Related Work

Multiatlas methods for segmentation, which were first introduced in [11, 18, 26], have become a very popular choice in medical image analysis due to their excellent performance. The methods have been extensively used on brain MR images [6, 12, 31], on cardiac CTA data [17], for thoracic CT segmentation [10, 33] and multiorgan segmentation in CT images [35]. Multiatlas methods generally produce robust results but rely on multiple image registrations as each atlas image is registered to the target image. Image registration can be divided into two different approaches: feature-based and intensity-based registrations, see the surveys [16, 28]. Feature-based methods are generally very fast, but may have a risk of failing due to many outlier correspondences between the images. The intensity-based methods are on the contrary capable of producing accurate registrations but may be slow and are sensitive to initialization.

Multiatlas segmentation is a further development from single-atlas segmentation [21] and works as follows. In order to capture more anatomical variations and reduce the effect of registration errors, several single-atlas segmentations are combined in the multiatlas approach. At first, pairwise registrations are computed between each atlas image and the target image, and thereafter, the single-atlas segmentation labels are transferred to the target image according to the registrations. Next, a segmentation proposal is obtained by fusing the transferred labels. The label fusion can be performed using several different methods, whereof the simplest one is majority voting for each voxel, see [11, 18, 26]. However, there exist more sophisticated methods, for instance weighted voting [32], probabilistic reasoning using, e.g. the STAPLE algorithm [34] and different types of machine-learning approaches [27]. The fused segmentation proposal can be further refined into a final segmentation by using graph cut [3, 22] or random forest-based methods [9]. For a comprehensive survey of multiatlas segmentation methods and their applications, see [13].

As mentioned previously, multiatlas methods are often used to perform multiorgan segmentation. In the work of Wolz et al. [35], a hierarchical atlas is refined at three levels: global, organ and voxel levels. Instead of utilizing all the available atlases, the authors choose the most suitable ones. Similar to our paper, their final segmentation is obtained using graph cuts, and the evaluation of the algorithm results in relatively high Dice index on the liver, kidneys, pancreas and spleen.

Another example of multiorgan segmentation is the probabilistic multiatlas used by Chu et al. [4] for abdominal segmentation. They divide the image space into N subspaces and compute weights for the probabilistic atlas at both for a global level ($N = 1$) and for each subspace. The organ segmentation is then obtained by a maximum a posteriori estimation and graph cuts. The method is evaluated on different numbers of subspaces, where the best performance is obtained for $N = 64$.

Furthermore, another variant of multiatlas segmentation of abdominal organs was used in a recent paper by Xu et al. [36]. Atlas selection and label fusion were done using a reformulation of the selective and iterative method for performance-level estimation (SIMPLE) method. The authors developed a method for atlas selection, which was regularized by a Bayesian prior, learnt from context information. When evaluating the proposed method, it outperformed the compared methods, among them [35], on 11 out of 12 organs.

In [23], Okada et al. present an approach to multiorgan segmentation that uses conditional shape-location combined with unsupervised intensity priors. In their work, an organ correlation graph is used to steer the order for which the organs are segmented by utilizing spatial correlation. In addition, the authors also developed a method for modelling conditional shape-location priors.

12.1.2   Our Approach

In this paper, we propose a pipeline for segmentation of 20 different organs in whole-body CT images. The algorithm uses standard multiatlas segmentation for initial spatial localization. For the pairwise registrations between the target image and all the atlas images, we use an adapted feature-based method that has been designed to reduce the risk of establishing incorrect point-to-point correspondences between the image pairs. The main contribution of this paper is a method to identify reliable organ-specific feature points among the atlas images. The speed of general feature-based registration methods is beneficial to the algorithm, especially since this identification is done in an offline preprocessing step. We fuse the transferred labels by training a random forest classifier, and the final segmentation is then obtained with graph cuts. The pipeline is described in detail in Sect. 12.2. In Sect. 12.3, we present the results from the VISCERAL Anatomy Challenge [15], as well as a detailed evaluation of the different steps in the pipeline for some of the organs.

12.2 Methods

Our pipeline for multiorgan segmentation contains the following three main steps:

1. *Pairwise Registration.* For a particular organ, the atlases are registered to the target image in two steps: first, *subsets* of the features in each atlas image are selected and matched to the features in the target image. Next, a non-rigid transformation between the atlases and the target image is estimated using RANSAC followed by a thin-plate spline (TPS) refinement or an intensity-based free-form deformation using NIFTYREG. See Sect. 12.2.1.
2. *Label Fusion with a Random Forest Classifier.* The pairwise registrations give us a rough estimate of the location of the target organ. However, the accuracy of the solution after the registration can be further improved by taking the local appearance surrounding the target organ into account. In order to do this, we train a random forest classifier that is used to fuse the transferred atlas labels after the registration. See Sect. 12.2.2.
3. *Graph Cut Segmentation with a Potts Model.* The segmentation is further refined by encouraging spatial smoothness between neighbouring pixels. For this, we formulate the labelling problem as an optimization problem and solve it using graph cuts. See Sect. 12.2.3.

These steps of our pipeline will be presented in detail in the following sections. Each organ is segmented individually in our multiatlas approach.

12.2.1 Pairwise Registration

12.2.1.1 Determination of Organ-Specific Feature Sets

For each organ and atlas image $I_i \in I = \{I_1, \ldots, I_n\}$, a subset of features that is designed to produce a reliable registration of the organ of interest is determined. The basic idea is to evaluate how well the extracted feature points in an atlas image match to other feature points in the remaining atlas images. In order to quantify the quality of a matched feature correspondence, we first establish the so-called golden transformations between the two atlas images around the organ of interest, based on precomputed (ground truth) landmark correspondences. Hence, if a feature point is matched to a feature point in another image, then this point-to-point correspondence should be consistent with the golden transformation, provided the correspondence is correct. Otherwise, it is likely to be an outlier. Feature points that always form inlier correspondences are good candidates for reliable registration, and these points determine the organ-specific feature sets.

Establishing golden transformations. For each atlas image, we compute golden transformations between I_i and the other atlas images in $I \setminus I_i$. This is done by applying TPS to precomputed landmark correspondences using the method proposed in [5]. The landmark correspondences are computed through accurate non-rigid registrations between a randomly chosen reference atlas in the atlas set and each of the remaining atlases. The registration uses two channels, the image intensity and the ground truth mask of the organ of interest, and maximizes the similarity between these according to the normalized mutual information (NMI) measure using NIFTYREG [1, 24]. With the obtained displacement field, the mesh points of a triangular mesh of the ground truth surfaces are transformed to the coordinate system of the reference atlas. For each mesh point (landmark) of the triangulation of the reference ground truth surface, the closest point on each transformed triangulated surface is found using an algorithm based on [8] and chosen as the corresponding landmark.

Feature extraction. For each atlas image, $I_i \in I$, we calculate sparse features according to the method proposed by Svärm et al. [29]. A feature point is denoted $\mathbf{f} = (i, \mathbf{x}, \mathbf{d})$ where i is the index of the image, and $\mathbf{x}$ and $\mathbf{d}$ are the coordinates and the description vector for the point, respectively. Only the features that lie sufficiently close to the organ are considered; that is, we keep features with distance to the organ, δ, less than a predefined threshold, $D_{\max}$. For the whole atlas I, we thus obtain $F = \{F_1, \dots, F_n\}$, where F_i is the set of feature points for I_i. For each atlas image I_i, the points in F_i are matched to the other feature sets in $F \setminus F_i$ using a symmetric neighbour approach, thus establishing point-to-point correspondences between I_i and the other atlas images.

Computation of organ-specific feature sets. Next, we proceed by applying the golden transformations to the feature points in $F \setminus F_i$ that have been matched to points in F_i, in order to transform them into the same coordinate system. Furthermore, we calculate the residuals between the coordinates of the feature points for I_i and the corresponding feature points for the other atlas images after the transformation. If feature point $\mathbf{f}_k \in F_i$ is matched to $\mathbf{f}_{\tilde{k}} \in F_j$, the residual is defined as

$$r_{\tilde{k}} = \|\mathbf{x}_k - \hat{\mathbf{T}}^G_{j,i} \circ \mathbf{x}_{\tilde{k}}\|_2, \tag{12.1}$$

where $\hat{\mathbf{T}}^G_{j,i}$ denotes the golden transformation between I_i and I_j. Each feature in F_i receives a score that is a weighted sum of the normalized residuals for all the corresponding points in the other atlas images and the normalized distance from the organ. More precisely, the score for $\mathbf{f}_k \in F_i$ is

$$\text{Score}[\mathbf{f}_k] = s_\delta + \omega_r \sum_{\tilde{k} \in \mathbf{R}} s_{\tilde{k}}, \tag{12.2}$$

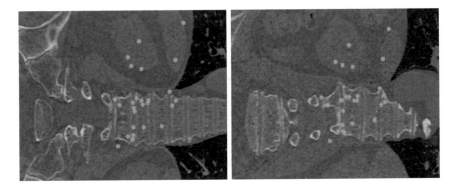

Fig. 12.1 Two CT slices of a target image (*left*) and an atlas image (*right*) with corresponding features after RANSAC for lumbar vertebra 1

where

$$s_\delta = (D_{\max} - \delta_k)/D_{\max},$$
$$s_{\tilde{k}} = \max(T - r_{\tilde{k}}, 0)/T. \qquad (12.3)$$

Here, ω_r is the importance weight for the residuals; T is a predefined threshold; and $\mathbf{R}$ is the set of feature points for the atlas images $I \setminus I_i$, which have been matched to $\mathbf{f}_k$. The features are ranked according to their score, and those with the highest scores are kept and used in the registration step. This procedure is relatively time-consuming, but it is an offline process and thus only done once.

12.2.1.2 Pairwise Registration with RANSAC

At run-time, we estimate pairwise affine transformations between the target image I_t and all the images in the atlas set, using the feature sets obtained in the previous section. We apply RANSAC with the truncated l_2 norm as a cost function for outlier removal. An example of inlier feature correspondences for the lumbar vertebra 1 is illustrated in Fig. 12.1. Furthermore, for about half of the organs, the final coordinate transforms between I and I_t are obtained by TPS interpolation between the remaining correspondences. For the rest of the organs, we find that the best transformations are obtained by using NIFTYREG, with the affine transformation as initialization. These transformations are then used to transfer the labels of the atlas images into the same coordinate system as the target image, see Fig. 12.2.

12.2.2 *Label Fusion with a Random Forest Classifier*

We use the pairwise registrations to obtain a rough estimate of where the organ is located. This is done by fusing the transferred labels from each atlas into a so-called

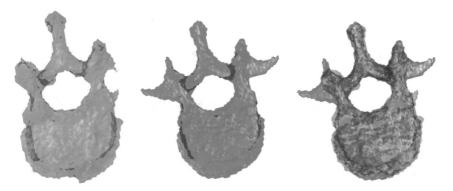

Fig. 12.2 Example of a registration of lumbar vertebra 1. *Left* the atlas ground truth mask. *Middle* the warped target mask after the registration. *Right* the masks overlaid in the same coordinate system

voxel map, P, in which each voxel can be interpreted as a measure of the likelihood of that voxel belonging to the organ, according to the pairwise registrations. More precisely, the map P is the normalized average of the warped target masks of each of the atlas images, so if half of the atlas images think that voxel i is organ, then $P(i) = 0.5$.

However, the map P largely ignores the local appearance around the target organ and in order to further improve the results, a random forest classifier is trained in an offline process. The classifier is then used to obtain a refined estimate of P, which will be denoted P_r. We implement this using Sherwood [7], which allows us to train and evaluate large random forest instances efficiently. The voxel map, P, and the target image, I, are used to compute a set of features for each voxel, which will be used as input to the random forest classifier. By smoothing I and P using a Gaussian kernel, we obtain two new volumes, which we refer to as I_s and P_s. Furthermore, for each organ we determine a threshold level, τ, for P and use this to construct a distance map, D_P, where each voxel in D_P equals the (signed) distance to the boundary surface of the binary volume $P > \tau$. For each voxel i, in each volume I, we thus obtain five features: $I(i)$, $I_s(i)$, $P(i)$, $P_s(i)$ and $D_P(i)$.

12.2.3   Graph Cut Segmentation with a Potts Model

The refined estimate, P_r, gives us a better estimation of the segmentation, but there is room for further improvement. The decision of whether voxel i should be classified as belonging to the organ or not is taken without considering the classification of neighbouring voxels, which may cause noisy and inaccurate estimates along the boundaries of the target organ. Thus, we can improve the segmentation by incorporating this information into the model, and in order to do so, we formulate our voxel labelling problem as an energy minimization problem and solve it using graph cuts [2]. More precisely, let $x_i \in \mathbf{L} = \{0, 1\}$ be a Boolean indicator variable for voxel i, that is, 1 if x_i is classified as belonging to the organ (foreground), and 0 if it belongs to the background. We are now seeking the labelling $\mathbf{x}^*$ that minimizes the energy function of the form

$$E(\mathbf{x}^*) = \sum_{i=1}^{n} D_i(x_i) + \sum_{i,j \in \mathbf{N}} V_{i,j}(x_i, x_j), \qquad (12.4)$$

where the data term, $D_i(x_i)$, measures how well the label x_i suits voxel i, given the target image I_t, and $V_{i,j}(x_i, x_j)$ is an interaction term that regularizes the solution by assigning different costs to neighbouring voxels, which depend on the labels they take. Furthermore, n is the number of voxels in the image, and $\mathbf{N}$ defines the neighbourhood system of the voxels.

The output from the random forest classifier is used for the data term, in which voxel i is set to take the value $1/2 - P_r(i)$ if $x_i = 1$, and zero otherwise, i.e. $D_i(x_i) = x_i(\frac{1}{2} - P_r(i))$. Thus, this model makes it more likely that voxel i is classified as foreground if $P_r(i) \in [0.5, 1]$, and background if $P_r(i) \in [0, 0.5]$. As interaction term, we use Potts model, which regularizes the resulting segmentation by penalizing neighbouring voxels if they receive different labels. It assigns a cost to two neighbouring voxels, i and j, according to $\lambda[x_i \neq x_j]$, where λ is a regularization weight, and x_i and x_j are the labels for voxels i and j, respectively. This interaction cost can also be expressed as $V_{i,j}(x_i, x_j) = \lambda(x_i(1 - x_j) + x_j(1 - x_i))$.

Thus, the final segmentation, $\mathbf{x}^*$, is obtained by solving the following minimization problem:

$$\mathbf{x}^* = \underset{\mathbf{x} \in \{0,1\}^n}{\operatorname{argmin}} \sum_{i=1}^{n} x_i \left(\frac{1}{2} - P_r(i)\right) + \lambda \sum_{i=1}^{n} \sum_{j \in \mathbf{N}(i)} \mu_{ij} x_i(1 - x_j), \qquad (12.5)$$

where μ_{ij} is a variable that compensates for anisotropic resolution [19], and $\mathbf{N}(i)$ is the set of voxels in the neighbourhood of voxel i, which is set to be 6-connected for all the organs, i.e. each voxel that touches a side of a voxel is a neighbour. Since the cost function in (12.5) is submodular, it can be minimized efficiently using graph cuts [20] with the implementation of [14]. During the minimization, we process a smaller volume, that is, a cut-out around the zero level of the thresholded voxel map $P > \tau$, which allows us to save memory and speed up the calculations.

A comparison between the resulting segmentation of the spleen with graph cuts, using the initial voxel map, P, and the refined probability map after the random forest step, P_r, is illustrated in Fig. 12.3.

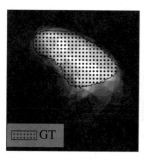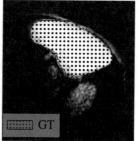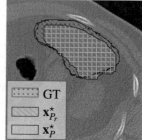

Fig. 12.3 Example of the resulting probability estimates and segmentation of the spleen for one CT slice; in each image, the ground truth (GT) is indicated. *Left* the initial probability, P. *Middle* the probability given by random forest, P_r. *Right* the resulting segmentation $\mathbf{x}_P^\star$ using P and $\mathbf{x}_{P_r}^\star$ using P_r overlaid on the original image

12.3 Experimental Evaluation

The different steps in the pipeline involve some tuning parameters and these have been set as follows. The 20 whole-body CT images that are available in the challenge are split into one training and validation (atlas) set consisting of the first 15 images, while the remaining five serve as a test set. For the registration, the parameters are determined by leave-one-out cross-validation of the atlas images, while the remaining ones are used as validation images for the random forest classification and graph cut segmentation.

For the computation of the organ-specific feature sets, the same parameter settings are used for all organs. At first, around 8,000–10,000 features are extracted from a whole-body CT image in less than 30 s. When ranking the features, the maximal distance is set to $D_{max} = 100$ mm, the threshold $T = 15$, and the importance weight for the residuals, ω, is set to 10. We have found empirically that the 300 features with the highest score can be used to provide robust and reliable registration. RANSAC is run 500,000 iterations, and the truncation threshold for the l_2 cost function is set to 30 mm. The value of the standard deviation, σ, for the Gaussian kernel in the smoothing of P for the random forest classifier is 1. Table 12.1 lists parameters and settings for each individual organ. Note that in the segmentation of some of the organs, we do not use a random forest classifier. This is either because the organ has a very large volume, which makes the computations heavy, or because the classifier does not improve the results at all. Furthermore, we do not use the learned features for the lungs. In our experience, very simple methods yield accurate segmentations of the lungs and that is also the case when we use ordinary features.

The single most time-consuming online part of the algorithm is the registration and the time needed strongly depends on the size of the organ and the choice of registration method. NIFTYREG takes around 100–200 s per registration compared to TPS for which a registration takes less than 10s regardless of the organ type. However, we have found empirically that NIFTYREG performs a lot better for ten of

Table 12.1 Parameters used in the pipeline

Organ	Registration method	RANSAC threshold	Random forest	τ	λ
Trachea	NIFTYREG	20	Yes	0.25	0.35
Right lung	TPS	30	No		0.35
Left lung	TPS	30	No		0.35
Pancreas	TPS	20	Yes	0.15	0.25
Gall bladder	TPS	25	No		0.15
Urinary bladder	TPS	50	Yes	1.45	0.35
Sternum	NIFTYREG	20	Yes	0.05	0.30
Lumbar vertebra 1	NIFTYREG	7	Yes	0.05	0.30
Right kidney	NIFTYREG	25	Yes	1.00	0.35
Left kidney	NIFTYREG	20	Yes	1.50	0.35
Right adrenal gland	TPS	30	No		0.20
Left adrenal gland	TPS	20	No		0.20
Right psoas major	NIFTYREG	40	Yes	0.45	0.40
Left psoas major	NIFTYREG	30	Yes	0.30	0.40
Muscle body of right rectus abdominis	NIFTYREG	40	Yes	0.05	0.30
Muscle body of left rectus abdominis	NIFTYREG	40	Yes	0.05	0.25
Aorta	NIFTYREG	30	Yes	0.20	0.35
Liver	TPS	50	Yes	0.90	0.40
Thyroid gland	TPS	20	Yes	0.10	0.25
Spleen	TPS	30	Yes	0.85	0.30

the organs, see Table 12.1. If more images are added to the training set, the process of determining the organ-specific features, the registration of the atlas images in order to obtain the voxel map, P, and the training of the random forest classifier would have to be run again from start. The only difference for the online process is that we would have to perform one extra registration per added image.

12.3.1 Challenge Results

In our contribution to the VISCERAL Anatomy Challenge, all the 20 images available for training formed the atlas set in the final submission. The algorithm was evaluated on a test set consisting of 10 new whole-body CT images that only were available to the organizers of the challenge, and the evaluation took place at ISBI 2015. The results are measured using the Dice index, which is defined as $\text{Dice}(S, G) = 2|S \cap G|/(|S| + |G|)$, where S and G are the computed segmentation and ground truth, respectively. Thus, a perfect segmentation would yield Dice index 1, while a segmentation with no ground truth overlap would receive a Dice index of

Table 12.2 Final results measured in Dice index for whole-body CT images. Here, "*" means that no segmentation was provided

Organ	Our	CMIV	HES-SO	SIAT
Left kidney	**0.934**	0.896	0.784	*
Right kidney	**0.915**	0.796	0.790	*
Spleen	0.870	**0.910**	0.703	0.874
Liver	0.921	**0.936**	0.866	0.923
Left lung	**0.972**	0.961	**0.972**	0.952
Right lung	**0.975**	0.970	**0.975**	0.957
Urinary bladder	**0.763**	0.713	0.698	*
Muscle body of left rectus abdominis	**0.746**	*	0.551	*
Muscle body of right rectus abdominis	**0.679**	*	0.519	*
Lumbar vertebra 1	**0.775**	*	0.718	*
Thyroid	0.424	*	**0.549**	*
Pancreas	0.383	*	**0.408**	*
Left psoas major muscle	**0.861**	0.828	0.806	*
Right psoas major muscle	**0.847**	0.817	0.787	*
Gall bladder	0.190	*	**0.276**	*
Sternum	**0.847**	*	0.761	*
Aorta	**0.830**	*	0.753	*
Trachea	**0.931**	*	0.92	*
Left adrenal gland	0.282	*	**0.373**	*
Right adrenal gland	0.220	*	**0.355**	*
Average	**0.718**	*	0.678	*

0. Our results are reported in Table 12.2 together with the results from the strongest participants:

- CMIV - "Centre for Medical Image Science and Visualization, Linköping University",
- HES-SO - "University of Applied Sciences Western Switzerland"
- SIAT - "Shenzhen Institutes of Advanced Technology, Chinese Academy of Sciences".

In summary, our algorithm provides the best results for 13 of the 20 organs.

12.3.2 Detailed Evaluation

In this section, we evaluate what kinds of benefits specific parts of the pipeline provide for lumbar vertebra 1, the left kidney and the spleen. Dice scores after

Table 12.3 Results for three organs after different steps in the pipeline, measured in Dice index. Here, OF indicates that ordinary feature sets were used instead of the organ-specific ones. $\mathbf{x}_P^\star$ is the map P, thresholded at τ and $\mathbf{x}^\star$ is the graph cut segmentation after the random forest step

Organ	$\mathbf{x}_P^\star$ (OF)	$\mathbf{x}^\star$ (OF)	$\mathbf{x}_P^\star$	$\mathbf{x}^\star$
Lumbar vertebra 1	0.730	0.682	0.858	0.884
Left kidney	0.891	0.901	0.891	0.896
Spleen	0.688	0.814	0.686	0.808

different steps in the pipeline, when using both organ-specific and ordinary feature sets, are presented in Table 12.3. We denote the segmentation that can be obtained after fusing the transferred labels from the registration with $\mathbf{x}_P^\star$ and it is the map P, thresholded at τ. The values in the table are the average results for the five images that formed the test set when using the 15 first as atlas set as described in the introduction to this section. Note that these values are not comparable with the ones in Table 12.2 since those were obtained with a different amount of training data and evaluated on images that are not accessible to us. The results in Table 12.3 should be compared among themselves in order to determine the contribution of different parts of the pipeline for the selected organs.

Clearly, the organ-specific features improve the results significantly for the segmentation of lumbar vertebra 1, which is demonstrated in Fig. 12.4. The left and the middle pictures in Fig. 12.5 show the segmentation of the spleen for CT image 19 before and after the graph cut part in the pipeline, respectively. It is clear from both the figures and the table that the random forest classifier improves the results a lot. However, note that the segmentation in the middle picture of Fig. 12.5 is not a valid spleen shape. The right picture of Fig. 12.5 illustrates the final segmentation for the left kidney. This segmentation is obtained using organ-specific features, and the result is quite accurate. However, the random forest classifier and the graph cut segmentation do not seem to further improve the Dice index for the left kidney according to the results in the table. Note that this does not necessarily mean that the segmentation is not improved. It is still possible that the produced solution is more regularized

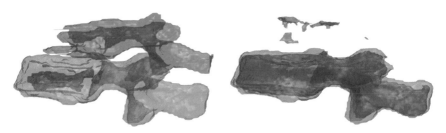

Fig. 12.4 Segmentation of lumbar vertebra 1. Here, the ground truth is *red* and our segmentation is *blue*. *Left* segmentation using ordinary features. The registration fails to find the correct vertebra as it is confused by a nearby vertebra. *Right* segmentation using organ-specific features. Now the correct vertebra is located

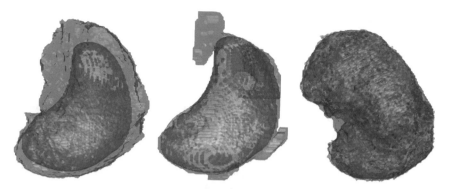

Fig. 12.5 Ground truth (*red*) and computed segmentation (*blue*) for some of the organs after different steps in the pipeline. Organ-specific features are used for all the segmentations. *Left* warped ground truth mask of the spleen after the registration. *Middle* graph cut segmentation of the spleen. *Right* graph cut segmentation of the *left* kidney

and accurate, just not according to the Dice index. Furthermore, the Dice scores for the left kidney and the spleen are more or less the same when using organ-specific features compared to when using ordinary features. In our experience, with a lot of training data the organ-specific features generally perform a little better than the ordinary features although that may not be the case for all the organs. It is, however, worth mentioning that there are certain limitations regarding the performance of the organ-specific features. It requires accurate landmark correspondences in order to establish reliable golden transformations, see Sect. 12.2.1. If this is not the case, it may not be advantageous to use organ-specific features.

12.4   Conclusions

In this paper, we have described an algorithm that uses a feature-based approach to multiatlas segmentation of organs in whole-body CT images. The results clearly demonstrate that this method manages to locate and segment the organs with the state-of-the-art results, and our approach outperforms the participants at the VISCERAL Anatomy Challenge on segmentation at ISBI 2015 for 13 out of 20 organs.

However, some parts of the algorithm could benefit from further work. For instance, incorporating prior information about the organ shapes into the pipeline would help to guarantee that the algorithm produces feasible organ shapes. A more thorough evaluation of the organ-specific feature sets could help determine individual parameter settings for the organs, as well as help in explaining why the method improves the results for some organs but not for all. Furthermore, adding additional features to the random forest classifier would likely yield better results. Moreover, the calculations could be sped up, e.g. by considering alternative registration methods.

References

1. Alvén J, Norlén A, Enqvist O, Kahl F (2016) Überatlas: fast and robust registration for multi-atlas segmentation. Pattern Recognit Lett. doi:10.1016/j.patrec.2016.05.001
2. Boykov Y, Veksler O, Zabih R (2001) Fast approximate energy minimization via graph cuts. IEEE Trans Pattern Anal Mach Intell 23(11):1222–1239
3. Candemir S, Jaeger S, Palaniappan K, Musco J, Singh R, Xue Z, Karargyris A, Antani S, Thoma G, McDonald C (2014) Lung segmentation in chest radiographs using anatomical atlases with nonrigid registration. IEEE Trans Med Imaging 33(2):577–590
4. Chu C, Oda M, Kitasaka T, Misawa K, Fujiwara M, Hayashi Y, Nimura Y, Rueckert D, Mori K (2013) Multi-organ segmentation based on spatially-divided probabilistic atlas from 3D abdominal CT images. In: Mori K, Sakuma I, Sato Y, Barillot C, Navab N (eds) MICCAI 2013. LNCS, vol 8150. Springer, Heidelberg, pp 165–172. doi:10.1007/978-3-642-40763-5_21
5. Chui H, Rangarajan A (2000) A new algorithm for non-rigid point matching. In: IEEE conference on computer vision and pattern recognition, vol 2, pp 44–51
6. Chupin M, Gérardin E, Cuingnet R, Boutet C, Lemieux L, Lehéricy S, Benali H, Garnero L, Colliot O (2009) Fully automatic hippocampus segmentation and classification in Alzheimer's disease and mild cognitive impairment applied on data from adni. Hippocampus 19(6):579–587
7. Criminisi A, Shotton J, Konukoglu E (2011) Decision forests: a unified framework for classification, regression, density estimation, manifold learning and semi-supervised learning. Found Trends® Comput Graph Vis 7:81–227
8. Eberly D (2008) Distance between point and triangle in 3D. Geometric Tools, LLC. http://www.geometrictools.com/
9. Han X (2013) Learning-boosted label fusion for multi-atlas auto-segmentation. In: Wu G, Zhang D, Shen D, Yan P, Suzuki K, Wang F (eds) MLMI 2013. LNCS, vol 8184. Springer, Cham, pp 17–24. doi:10.1007/978-3-319-02267-3_3
10. Han X, Hoogeman MS, Levendag PC, Hibbard LS, Teguh DN, Voet P, Cowen AC, Wolf TK (2008) Atlas-based auto-segmentation of head and neck CT images. In: Metaxas D, Axel L, Fichtinger G, Székely G (eds) MICCAI 2008. LNCS, vol 5242. Springer, Heidelberg, pp 434–441. doi:10.1007/978-3-540-85990-1_52
11. Heckemann RA, Hajnal JV, Aljabar P, Rueckert D, Hammers A (2006) Automatic anatomical brain MRI segmentation combining label propagation and decision fusion. NeuroImage 33(1):115–126
12. Heckemann RA, Keihaninejad S, Aljabar P, Rueckert D, Hajnal JV, Hammers A (2010) Improving intersubject image registration using tissue-class information benefits robustness and accuracy of multi-atlas based anatomical segmentation. Neuroimage 51(1):221–227
13. Iglesias JE, Sabuncu MR (2015) Multi-atlas segmentation of biomedical images: a survey. Med Image Anal 24(1):205–219
14. Jamriška O, Sýkora D, Hornung A (2012) Cache-efficient graph cuts on structured grids. In: IEEE conference on computer vision and pattern recognition, pp 3673–3680
15. Jiménez-del-Toro OA, Müller H, Krenn M, Gruenberg K, Taha AA, Winterstein M, Eggel I, Foncubierta-Rodríguez A, Goksel O, Jakab A, Kontokotsios G, Langs G, Menze B, Fernandez TS, Schaer R, Walleyo A, Weber M, Cid YD, Gass T, Heinrich M, Jia F, Kahl F, Kechichian R, Mai D, Spanier AB, Vincent G, Wang C, Wyeth D, Hanbury A (2016) Cloud-based evaluation of anatomical structure segmentation and landmark detection algorithms: VISCERAL anatomy benchmarks. IEEE Trans Med Imaging 35(11):2459–2475
16. Khalifa F, Beache G, Gimel'farb G, Suri J, El-Baz A (2011) State-of-the-art medical image registration methodologies: a survey. In: El-Baz AS, Rajendra Acharya U, Mirmehdi M, Suri JS (eds) Multi modality state-of-the-art medical image segmentation and registration methodologies. Springer, Heidelberg, pp 235–280
17. Kirisli HA, Schaap M, Klein S, Neefjes LA, Weustink AC, van Walsum T, Niessen WJ (2010) Fully automatic cardiac segmentation from 3D CTA data: a multi-atlas based approach. In: SPIE medical imaging, San Diego, USA

18. Klein A, Mensh B, Ghosh S, Tourville J, Hirsch J (2005) Mindboggle: automated brain labeling with multiple atlases. BMC Med Imaging 5(1):7
19. Kolmogorov V, Boykov Y (2005) What metrics can be approximated by geo-cuts, or global optimization of length/area and flux. In: IEEE international conference on computer vision, vol 1, pp 564–571
20. Kolmogorov V, Zabin R (2004) What energy functions can be minimized via graph cuts? IEEE Trans Pattern Anal Mach Intell 26(2):147–159
21. Kurkure U, Le Y, Ju T, Carson J, Paragios N, Kakadiaris I (2011) Subdivision-based deformable model for geometric atlas fitting. In: IEEE international conference on computer vision, Barcelona, Spain
22. Lee JG, Gumus S, Moon CH, Kwoh CK, Bae KT (2014) Fully automated segmentation of cartilage from the MR images of knee using a multi-atlas and local structural analysis method. Med Phys 41(9)
23. Okada T, Linguraru MG, Hori M, Summers RM, Tomiyama N, Sato Y (2015) Abdominal multi-organ segmentation from CT images using conditional shape-location and unsupervised intensity priors. Med Image Anal 26(1):1–18
24. Ourselin S, Roche A, Subsol G, Pennec X, Ayache N (2001) Reconstructing a 3D structure from serial histological sections. Image Vis Comput 19(1–2):25–31
25. Pekar V, McNutt TR, Kaus MR (2004) Automated model-based organ delineation for radiotherapy planning in prostatic region. Int J Radiat Oncol Biol Phys 60(3):973–980
26. Rohlfing T, Brandt R, Menzel R, Maurer CR Jr (2004) Evaluation of atlas selection strategies for atlas-based image segmentation with application to confocal microscopy images of bee brains. NeuroImage 21(4):1428–1442
27. Sanroma G, Wu G, Gao Y, Shen D (2014) Learning-based atlas selection for multiple-atlas segmentation. In: IEEE conference on computer vision and pattern recognition, Columbus, USA
28. Sotiras A, Davatzikos C, Paragios N (2013) Deformable medical image registration: a survey. IEEE Trans Med Imaging 32(7):1153–1190
29. Svärm L, Enqvist O, Kahl F, Oskarsson M (2015) Improving robustness for inter-subject medical image registration using a feature-based approach. In: International symposium on biomedical imaging
30. Taylor R, Stoianovici D (2003) Medical robotics in computer-integrated surgery. IEEE Trans Robot Autom 19(5):765–781
31. van der Lijn F, den Heijer T, Breteler MM, Niessen WJ (2008) Hippocampus segmentation in MR images using atlas registration, voxel classification, and graph cuts. NeuroImage 43(4):708–720
32. Wang H, Suh J, Dass SR, Pluta J, Craige C, Yushkevich P (2013) Multi-atlas segmentation with joint label fusion. IEEE Trans Pattern Anal Mach Intell 35(3):611–623
33. Wang L, Chen KC, Gao Y, Shi F, Liao S, Li G, Shen SGF, Yan J, Lee PKM, Chow B, Liu NX, Xia JJ, Shen D (2014) Automated bone segmentation from dental CBCT images using patch-based sparse representation and convex optimization. Med Phys 41(4):043503
34. Warfield S, Zou K, Wells W (2004) Simultaneous truth and performance level estimation (STAPLE): an algorithm for the validation of image segmentation. IEEE Trans Med Imaging 27(3):903–921
35. Wolz R, Chu C, Misawa K, Fujiwara M, Mori K, Rueckert D (2013) Automated abdominal multi-organ segmentation with subject-specific atlas generation. IEEE Trans Med Imaging 32(9):1723–1730
36. Xu Z, Burke RP, Lee CP, Baucom RB, Poulose BK, Abramson RG, Landman BA (2015) Efficient multi-atlas abdominal segmentation on clinically acquired CT with SIMPLE context learning. Med Image Anal 24(1):18–27

Part V
VISCERAL Retrieval Participant Reports

Chapter 13
Combining Radiology Images and Clinical Metadata for Multimodal Medical Case-Based Retrieval

Oscar Jimenez-del-Toro, Pol Cirujeda and Henning Müller

Abstract As part of their daily workload, clinicians examine patient cases in the process of formulating a diagnosis. These large multimodal patient datasets stored in hospitals could help in retrieving relevant information for a differential diagnosis, but these are currently not fully exploited. The VISCERAL Retrieval Benchmark organized a medical case-based retrieval algorithm evaluation using multimodal (text and visual) data from radiology reports. The common dataset contained patient CT (Computed Tomography) or MRI (Magnetic Resonance Imaging) scans and RadLex term anatomy–pathology lists from the radiology reports. A content-based retrieval method for medical cases that uses both textual and visual features is presented. It defines a weighting scheme that combines the anatomical and clinical correlations of the RadLex terms with local texture features obtained from the region of interest in the query cases. The visual features are computed using a 3D Riesz wavelet texture analysis performed on a common spatial domain to compare the images in the analogous anatomical regions of interest in the dataset images. The proposed method obtained the best mean average precision in 6 out of 10 topics and the highest number of relevant cases retrieved in the benchmark. Obtaining robust results for various pathologies, it could further be developed to perform medical case-based retrieval on large multimodal clinical datasets.

O. Jimenez-del-Toro (✉) · H. Müller
Institute of Information Systems, University of Applied Sciences Western Switzerland
Sierre (HES-SO), Sierre, Switzerland
e-mail: oscar.jimenez@hevs.ch

H. Müller
University Hospitals of Geneva, Geneva, Switzerland
e-mail: henning.mueller@hevs.ch

P. Cirujeda
Department of Information and Communication Technologies,
Universitat Pompeu Fabra, Barcelona, Spain
e-mail: pol.cirujeda@upf.edu

© The Author(s) 2017
A. Hanbury et al. (eds.), *Cloud-Based Benchmarking
of Medical Image Analysis*, DOI 10.1007/978-3-319-49644-3_13

221

13.1   Introduction

As part of their daily workload, clinicians have to visualize and interpret a large number of medical images and radiology reports [17]. In recent years, the volume of images in medical records has increased due to the continuous development of imaging modalities and storage capabilities in hospitals [18]. Going through these large amounts of data is time-consuming and not scalable with the current trend of big data analysis [16]. Therefore, the challenge to make an efficient use of these large datasets and to provide useful information for the diagnostic decisions of clinicians is of high relevance [19]. It is of particular significance to effectively combine the information contained both in the patients' medical imaging and the clinical metadata from their reports [14].

It is now common for research groups to test their retrieval algorithms on a private dataset, impeding the repeatability of their results and comparison to other algorithms [7]. The Visual Concept Extraction Challenge in Radiology (VISCERAL) project was developed as a cloud-based infrastructure for the evaluation of medical image analysis techniques on large datasets [16]. Through evaluation campaigns, challenges, benchmarks and competitions, tasks of general interest can be selected to compare the algorithms on a large scale. One of these tasks is the Retrieval Benchmark, which aims to find cases with similar anomalies based on query cases [11].

In this paper, a multimodal (text and visual) approach for medical case-based retrieval is presented. It uses the RadLex [15] terminology and the 3D texture features extracted from medical images to objectively compare and rank the relevance of medical cases for a differential diagnosis. Via an estimation of anatomical regions of interest in the spatial domain delineated in medical images, it exploits the visual similarities in the 3D patient scans to improve the baseline text rankings [10]. The implementation of the method, set up and results in the VISCERAL Retrieval Benchmark and lessons learned are explained in the following sections.

13.2   Materials and Methods

The proposed approach to retrieve relevant medical cases was based on a weighting score scheme that combined RadLex terms' anatomical and pathological correlations with local visual information.

The VISCERAL Retrieval dataset on which this method was implemented and tested is initially addressed. The clinical metadata weighting scheme is then explained. Afterwards, the various image processing techniques used for the visual feature extraction approach are shown. Finally, the fusion of both data, RadLex term lists and 3D patient scans, is explained in the multimodal fusion section.

13.2.1 Dataset

The Retrieval benchmark dataset was composed of patient scans (3D volumes) and RadLex anatomy–pathology term lists. The 2311 images in the dataset were obtained during clinical routine from two data providers.[1] The dataset had a heterogeneous collection of images including computed tomography (CT) and magnetic resonance imaging (MRI) T1- and T2-weighted imaging, enhanced and unenhanced, in different fields of view (e.g. abdomen, whole body). For 1813 cases, RadLex anatomy–pathology term lists were generated automatically from the radiology reports of the images. They included the affected anatomical structures and their RadLex term ID, the pathologies and their Radlex term ID, and whether the findings were negated or not in the report. The number of findings and anatomical structures involved varied from case to case.

13.2.2 VISCERAL Retrieval Benchmark Evaluation Setup

Ten query topics, not included in the dataset, were distributed to the participants for the evaluation of their retrieval algorithms. The goal of the benchmark was to detect and rank relevant cases in the dataset that could potentially aid in the process of diagnosing the query cases. Each query topic was composed of the following data:

- List of RadLex anatomy–pathology terms from the radiology report
- 3D patient scan (CT or MRT1/MRT2)
- Manually annotated 3D mask of the main organ affected
- Manually annotated 3D region of interest (ROI) from the radiologist's perspective

Participants submitted their rankings and medical experts performed relevance judgements on the submitted cases to determine if they were relevant for the diagnosis of each of the query topics.

13.2.3 Multimodal Medical Case Retrieval

13.2.3.1 Text Retrieval

Given a set of N medical cases $C = \langle \mathbf{R}_1, \ldots, \mathbf{R}_N; \mathbf{V}_1, \ldots, \mathbf{V}_N; \mathbf{M}_1, \ldots, \mathbf{M}_N; \mathbf{F}_1, \ldots, \mathbf{F}_N \rangle$ where the textual information from a radiological report $\mathbf{R}_n$ contains a list L of the anatomies A and pathologies P present in the medical case $\mathbf{C}_n$. The visual information $(\mathbf{V}_n, \mathbf{M}_n, \mathbf{F}_n)$ includes a triple of 3D volumes, containing the patient volume $\mathbf{V}_n$, binary label organ mask (annotation) $\mathbf{M}_n$ and binary label region of interest (annotation) $\mathbf{F}_n$.

---

[1]http://www.visceral.eu/benchmarks/retrieval-benchmark/, as of 15 July 2016.

The aim is to create a ranking S of relevant cases $\mathscr{S} = \langle \mathbf{C}^1, \ldots \mathbf{C}^S \rangle$ useful for a differential diagnosis with the target case $\mathbf{C}_T$. Each case $\mathbf{C}_n$ is evaluated according to its radiology report $\mathbf{R}_n$ and visual information $(\mathbf{V}_n, \mathbf{M}_n, \mathbf{F}_n)$, and a final score A ranks the set of cases according to their relevance weight w.

$$\mathbf{S}'_T = (\mathbf{C}_1(w_1), \mathbf{C}_2(w_2), \ldots, \mathbf{C}_n(w_n)) \tag{13.1}$$

The correlations were computed with the RadLex term lists provided from the radiology reports. Each similarity feature had a different weight in the final decision for the differential diagnosis and retrieval of cases. The textual similarity between two cases was computed according to the following correlations and their correspondent weighting score (in brackets):

1. Same anatomy with same pathology [0.6]
2. Same anatomy with same pathology negated [0.55]
3. Same anatomy present multiple times [0.2]
4. Same anatomy mentioned once [0.1]
5. Same pathology with different anatomy [0.05]
6. Similar anatomies [0.05]
7. Same imaging modality [0.02]

The similarity features were defined using a heuristic approach, after a medical expert reviewed a subset of the RadLex term lists from randomly selected cases in the Retrieval dataset. The selected criteria were optimized on the subset cases and the clinical expertise of the medical expert. The aim of the weightings is to identify and highlight clinical features that could be relevant for a differential diagnosis and incorporate a priori knowledge of the types of image scans contained in the dataset. The ranking was performed by adding all the weights from the different similarity features for each case based on their corresponding RadLex term list. An independent score was generated for each case in the Retrieval dataset. To define similar anatomies, a list of correlating RadLex terms (e.g. lung, superior lobe, pleura...) was manually generated by a medical expert from the standard RadLex term hierarchy on the subset of randomly selected cases.[2] These lists were generated for each of the query topics in the benchmark.

13.2.3.2 Helping Multimodal Retrieval with Visual Texture Features

Multimodal retrieval can be influenced by common image processing techniques used in template matching or visual likelihood metrics for content-based image retrieval. Computer vision research areas such as image classification and pattern recognition from visible features such as colour, contours or texture have been present in recent approaches for the retrieval of medical cases with likely affected organs, image modalities or diagnosis [6].

---

[2]http://www.RadLex.org, as of 15 July 2016.

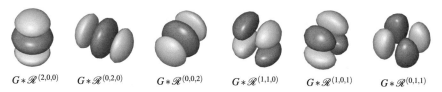

$G * \mathscr{R}^{(2,0,0)}$ $G * \mathscr{R}^{(0,2,0)}$ $G * \mathscr{R}^{(0,0,2)}$ $G * \mathscr{R}^{(1,1,0)}$ $G * \mathscr{R}^{(1,0,1)}$ $G * \mathscr{R}^{(0,1,1)}$

Fig. 13.1 Second-order Riesz kernels $\mathscr{R}^{(n_1,n_2,n_3)}$ convolved with isotropic Gaussian kernels $G(\boldsymbol{x})$

This section defines a methodology for content-based image retrieval via a similarity measurement from texture-based visual cues. First, a region of interest from a query image is characterized, thanks to its computed 3D Riesz wavelet coefficients. In order to deal with 3D structure and also to provide a more compact representation, these features are translated into a particular descriptor space which arises from modelling the covariance matrices of the coefficient observations within a volumetric region, instead of keeping the whole set of feature values. This compact data representation is of crucial interest as it allows to translate both learning image templates and unknown testing image candidates to a common space which can be used in a dictionary-seeking fashion for visual-based retrieval.

13.2.3.3   3D Riesz Transform for Texture Features

Riesz filterbanks are used in order to characterize the 3D texture of regions of interest in CT images. In previous work, 3D Riesz wavelets have demonstrated successful performance in the modelling task of subtle local 3D texture properties with high reproducibility compared to other methods [8, 9].

The Nth order Riesz transform $\mathscr{R}^{(N)}$ of a three-dimensional signal $f(\boldsymbol{x})$ is defined in the Fourier frequency domain as:

$$\widehat{\mathscr{R}^{(n_1,n_2,n_3)}f}(\boldsymbol{\omega}) = \sqrt{\frac{n_1 + n_2 + n_3}{n_1! n_2! n_3!}} \frac{(-j\omega_1)^{n_1}(-j\omega_2)^{n_2}(-j\omega_3)^{n_3}}{||\boldsymbol{\omega}||^{n_1+n_2+n_3}} \hat{f}(\boldsymbol{\omega}), \qquad (13.2)$$

for all combinations of (n_1, n_2, n_3) with $n_1 + n_2 + n_3 = N$ and $n_{1,2,3} \in \mathbb{N}$. Equation 13.2 yields $\binom{N+2}{2}$ templates $\mathscr{R}^{(n_1,n_2,n_3)}$ and forms multi-scale filterbanks when coupled with a multi-resolution framework.

In order to achieve a three-dimensional representation, the second-order Riesz filterbank (depicted in Fig. 13.1) is used and rotation invariance is obtained by locally aligning the Riesz components $\mathscr{R}^{(n_1,n_2,n_3)}$ of all scales based on the locally prevailing orientation as presented in [3].

13.2.3.4   Invariant Representation via 3D Covariance Descriptors

The choice of a particular set of features for an accurate texture description is as important as a representation that is able to yield invariance to scale, rotation or other spatial changes of the described region of interest. Riesz features are used in conjunction with a representation that takes into account their statistical distribution, leading to a compact and discriminative notation with several benefits for pattern recognition.

First, a spatial homogenization baseline is achieved by an indirect 3D spatial registration, where a reference image is used to register all the images from the dataset and generate a common space domain for visual comparison. The reference image is obtained from a control case of a complete patient scan in order to provide a complete alignment frame. Once a new image is provided as a query, it is first registered to the reference image and included in this rough alignment of the dataset images. Then, a set of derived regions of interest is determined for each of the images in the dataset by directly transforming the same coordinates from the ROI in the query image. See Fig. 13.2 for a scheme of this workflow.

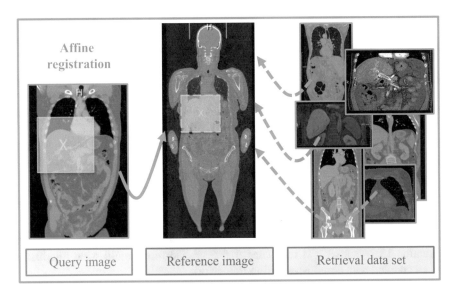

Fig. 13.2 Finding the region of interest (ROI) from the query image in the dataset. The image with the biggest size from the dataset was selected as the reference image. In order to have a common spatial domain to compare the images, all the images from the dataset were registered in advance to this reference image using affine registration (*dashed blue arrows*). With a new query, the query images were also registered to the reference image, and the provided binary mask for the ROI (*yellow borders*) was transformed using the coordinate transformation from the affine registration of the query image. This procedure defined an indirect ROI (*dashed yellow borders*) in each of the dataset images to compare the visual similarities with the query image

The required registrations for this step were computed using the image registration implementation from the Elastix software[3] [13]. The quality of the registration is iteratively evaluated in each optimization of a cost function that aims to minimize the normalized cross correlation from the voxel intensities of the transformed moving image to the fixed target image. Using affine registration, the 3D volumes are globally aligned through an iterative stochastic gradient descent optimizer with a multi-resolution approach [12].

The steerability property [21] of Riesz features asserts that voxel intensity values are projected to the direction of maximum variability within the region of interest, thus providing a common reference space for all the observable tissue patterns. Therefore, features are guaranteed to be directionality invariant which, added to the rotation-invariant representation explained below, adds an additional robustness to spatial changes in the proposed covariance descriptor framework.

By their construction, covariance descriptors are suitable for unstructured, abstract texture characterization inside a region, regardless of spatial rigid transformations such as rotation, scale or translations [2]. This is due to a statistics-based representation in which covariance is used as a measure of how several random variables change together (3D Riesz texture features in this case) and used as a discriminative signature of a region of interest. This notion translates the absolute feature space, which is sparse and high dimensional, to a meaningful lower dimensional space of feature covariances where regions with similar texture variabilities lie clustered and differentiated. Furthermore, the construction of covariance descriptors in their natural shape as symmetric positive definite matrices adds an inherent analytical methodology: these matrices form a manifold which can be analysed by its own defined Riemannian metrics [1] for the comparison of descriptor samples.

In order to formally define the 3D Riesz-covariance descriptors, a feature selection function $\Phi(ct, v)$ is denoted for a given 3D CT volume v (in this approach, a single $96 \times 96 \times 96$ block generated using the centre of the bounding box surrounding the manually annotated mask of the main organ affected in each the query topics) as:

$$\Phi(v) = \left\{ \mathcal{R}_{x,y,z}^{(n_1,n_2,n_3)}, \ \forall x, y, z \in v \right\}, \tag{13.3}$$

which denotes the set of 6-dimensional Riesz feature vectors, as defined in Eq. 13.2, obtained at each one of the coordinates $\{x, y, z\}$ contained in the volume cube v.

Then, for a given region v of the CT image, the associated covariance descriptor can be obtained as:

$$Cov(\Phi(v)) = \frac{1}{N-1} \sum_{i=1}^{N} (\Phi - \mu)(\Phi - \mu)^T, \tag{13.4}$$

where μ is the vector mean of the set of feature vectors $\{\Phi_{x,y,z}\}$ within the volumetric neighbourhood made of $N = 96^3$ samples. Figure 13.3 shows the construction of a sample 3D Riesz-covariance descriptor.

---

[3]http://elastix.isi.uu.nl, as of 20th October 2015.

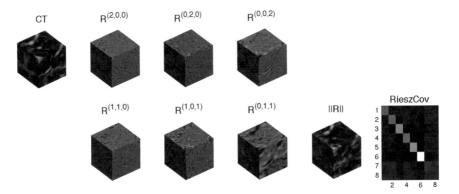

Fig. 13.3 Cues involved in the descriptor calculation for a given CT cubic region. The initial cube depicts the values within a $96 \times 96 \times 96$ pixel volume with its CT intensities; the 6 central cubes depict the 2nd order 3D-Riesz wavelet responses, and the Riesz norm is included as well. The matrix in the right sub-figure depicts the resulting covariance descriptor, encoding the different correlations between the distributions of the observed cues

13.2.3.5   Pattern Matching in the Sym_d^+ Manifold

The resulting 6×6 covariance descriptors are symmetric matrices in which the diagonal elements represent the variance of each Riesz feature, and the non-diagonal elements represent their pairwise covariance. As previously stated, these descriptors are used as discriminative signatures of the texture patterns found in the block v. 3D Riesz-based covariance descriptors do not only provide a representative entity, but they also lie in the Riemannian manifold of symmetric definite positive matrices Sym_d^+. The spatial distribution of the descriptor space is geometrically meaningful as 3D regions sharing similar texture characteristics remain clustered when descriptor similarity is computed by means of the Riemannian metrics defined for this non-Euclidean spatial distribution, as defined below. This is depicted in Fig. 13.4, where multi-dimensional scaling is used for projecting the descriptor space into a two-dimensional plot for visualization. The same notion can be used for feature selection or dimensionality reduction in the nonlinear descriptor space.

According to [1], the Sym_d^+ Riemannian manifold constituting the covariance descriptor space can be approximated in close neighbourhoods by the Euclidean metric in its tangent space, T_Y, where the symmetric matrix Y is a reference projection point in the manifold. T_Y is formed by a vector space of $d \times d$ symmetric matrices, and the tangent mapping of a manifold element X to $x \in T_Y$ is made by the point-dependent $\log_Y$ operation:

$$x = \log_Y(X) = Y^{\frac{1}{2}} \log \left(Y^{-\frac{1}{2}} X Y^{-\frac{1}{2}} \right) Y^{\frac{1}{2}}. \tag{13.5}$$

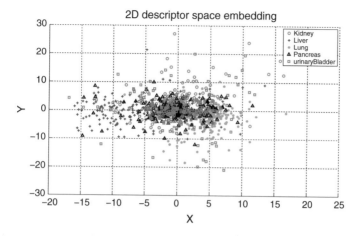

Fig. 13.4 Set of image descriptors obtained from 5 organ textures, belonging to 200 different cubic samples from various patient CT scans. The descriptors for each class are plotted in different colours in the embedded two-dimensional space, via the multi-dimensional scaling dimensionality reduction technique, according to the descriptor similarity metric defined in Eq. 13.8. This plot demonstrates geometrical coherence as the class distribution is correlated in the descriptor space: areas with different texture features, such as liver, lung or urinary bladder, appear clustered in the descriptor space. Some areas that share texture features, such as pancreas appear more overlapped to other regions. In any case, this descriptor space can be used in linear or nonlinear machine learning classification methods for texture modelling

As a computational approximation in certain classification problems, the projection point can be established in a common point such as the Identity matrix, and therefore, the tangent mapping becomes:

$$\log(X) = U\log(D)U',$$ (13.6)

where U and D are the elements of the single value decomposition (SVD) of $X \in Sym_d^+$.

One property of the projected symmetric matrices in the tangent space T_Y is that they contain only $d(d + 1)/2$ independent coefficients, in their upper or lower triangular parts. Therefore, it is possible to apply the vectorization operation in order to obtain a linear orthonormal space for the independent coefficients:

$$\hat{x} = vect(x) = (x_{1,1}, x_{1,2}, \ldots, x_{1,d}, x_{2,2}, x_{2,3}, \ldots, x_{d,d}),$$ (13.7)

where x is the mapping of $X \in Sym_d^+$ to the tangent space, resulting from Eq. 13.5. The obtained vector $\hat{x}$ lies in the Euclidean space $\mathbb{R}^m$, where $m = d(d + 1)/2$. This can be used for efficient template storage in cases of big data volumes.

This set of operations is useful for data visualization, feature selection and for developing machine learning and classification techniques on top of the particular geometric space of the proposed covariance descriptors. The tangent mapping operator can be taken into account leading to the following Riemannian metric, which expresses the geodesic distance between two points X_1 and X_2 on Sym_d^+ [1]:

$$\delta(X_1, X_2) = \sqrt{Trace\left(\log\left(X_1^{-\frac{1}{2}} X_2 X_1^{-\frac{1}{2}}\right)^2\right)}, \qquad (13.8)$$

or more simply $\delta(X_1, X_2) = \sqrt{\sum_{i=1}^{d} \log(\lambda_i)^2}$, where λ_i are the positive eigenvalues of $X_1^{-\frac{1}{2}} X_2 X_1^{-\frac{1}{2}}$.

Therefore, in a similarity retrieval application in which a query region obtained covariance descriptor Q has to be matched against a set of template region descriptors $\{T_i\}$ belonging to different classes, this distance can be used as a supporting metric for a weighted scoring system for multimodal retrieval:

$$class(Q) = \underset{i}{\operatorname{argmin}} \{\delta(Q, T_i) \, \forall i \in T\}, \qquad (13.9)$$

since the dimensionality of the proposed descriptors is very compact, this scoring function is computationally feasible for datasets of reasonable sizes.

13.2.3.6 Multimodal Fusion

It is known from previous medical case-based retrieval benchmarks that the text queries obtain much better results than the visual queries [4, 5]. This has been attributed to the currently much more consistent representation of clinical signs in medical images by text labels than by their visual features that are not always very specific. Therefore, it is of high interest to the retrieval information community to find robust visual features that can be combined with semantic terms [14]. To include the information obtained from the visual ranking of the cases into the semantic text weighting scheme, we give an additional weighting if the visual similarity score is high. The additional weight [0.05] is added to the total sum from the textual score of the case, if it is in the top 20% of the ranking obtained from the similarity score of the covariance descriptor. These parameters were manually optimized using a small subset of the dataset. A medical expert provided a list of correlation-based similarities that are of interest for finding relevant cases in the dataset. For each of the query topics, a single main combination of anatomy and pathology RadLex terms was manually selected from RadLex term list. This decision was based on the region of interest and organ mask provided in the benchmark to the participants.

13.3 Results

Only one run was submitted for the VISCERAL Retrieval benchmark 2015, which combined both the RadlexID weighting score scheme and the visual texture features. This run contained a ranking of 300 cases for each of the ten query topics in the benchmark. The cases were ranked in descending order according to the computed similarity to the query topic.

The proposed approach obtained the highest mean average precision (MAP) scores in 6 out of the 10 query topics [11]. The topic with the highest MAP was topic 08—kidney cyst—with 0.5131, and the lowest was topic 10—rib fracture—with 0.0467. The mean MAP was 0.2367 which was the second best MAP score of the benchmark.

Although the precision from 10 (P_10), 20 (P_20) and 30 (P_30) documents retrieved is lower than the method by Spanier et al. [20], our method presented a more stable decline of precision scores obtaining the benchmark top scores for 100 (P_100) and 200 (P_200) documents retrieved (see Fig. 13.5). Moreover, the proposed method obtained the highest total of relevant documents retrieved (num_rel_ret): 1077 out of a maximum of 2462. In 7 of the 10 query topics, it obtained the top number of total documents retrieved out of all the different 21 runs in the benchmark (see Fig. 13.6). The mean average precision (MAP), precision after query relevant cases retrieved (Rprec), binary preference (bpref), precision after 10 cases retrieved (P_10) and precision after 30 cases retrieved (P_30) from our method are shown per query topic in Table 13.1. These results take special interest when compared against the other retrieval methods proposed in order to identify which components receive a particular benefit when a multimodal-based scoring is introduced. There is a clear advantage of the method by Spanier et al. in query topic 10 when compared to our method. This topic, with radiological diagnosis of rib fracture, had only 47 cases

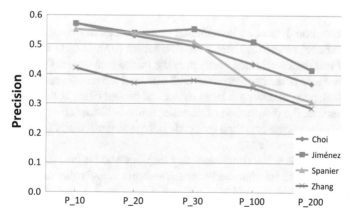

Fig. 13.5 Line graph showing the mean precision scores over all the topics at varying number of cases retrieved: 10–200. The best run was selected per participant considering all possible techniques: only text, only visual or mixed. A maximum of 300 cases could be included in each of the submitted rankings per topic

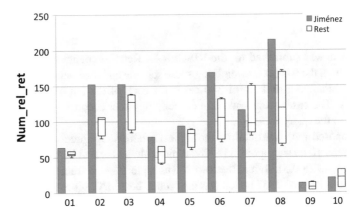

Fig. 13.6 Box plot chart with the total number of relevant cases retrieved (num_rel_ret) per topic in the VISCERAL Retrieval benchmark. The method proposed in this paper is represented with *red solid bars*. The results of the other participants, including text, visual and mixed runs are shown as *white boxes*. The *horizontal lines* inside the boxes mark the median number of relevant cases retrieved. Each box extends from the first to the third quantile of the run results

considered as relevant by the relevance judgements. This is one of the topics in the Retrieval Benchmark with fewer relevant cases, making it harder to select only a few relevant cases from the complete dataset. On the other hand, our method was the only run with a mixed technique (text and visual) that produced a ranking for all of the query topics available, unlike the approach from Spanier et al.

13.3.1 Lessons Learned

Having a common dataset is fundamental to make objective comparisons between different retrieval methods. There were two topics (07 and 09), where techniques using only text data performed better than the mixed techniques. Otherwise, multi-modal techniques in the benchmark overall obtained the best scores.

An advantage of scanning a large dataset of patient cases is that, like in a real clinical scenario, the distribution of diseases is not uniform. This requires a robust selection of relevant features for a successful retrieval, particularly for those diseases with few cases in the dataset.

Visual retrieval is still a complementary technique that is best used with a strong baseline of text-related similarities between medical cases. Further research is needed to detect the most relevant region of interest in the images as well as the best visual features per topic. Manual annotation of the regions of interest in the medical images can be useful to improve even further this technique by obtaining more targeted visual features related to a specific medical case. This would avoid sampling large regions in the image and generate a more robust training set on which to build

Table 13.1 Results for the 10 query topics in the VISCERAL Retrieval benchmark using the proposed multimodal (text and visual) retrieval approach

Metric	01	02	03	04	05	06	07	08	09	10	All
MAP	0.2293	0.2227	0.2227	0.2497	0.1949	0.3883	0.1780	0.5131	0.1212	0.0467	**0.2367**
Rprec	0.4576	0.3575	0.3575	0.3106	0.3508	0.4985	0.3483	0.6399	0.1667	0.0851	**0.3572**
bpref	0.5035	0.3466	0.3466	0.4047	0.3542	0.4912	0.3444	0.6307	0.1580	0.0837	**0.3664**
P10	0.2000	0.6000	0.6000	0.8000	0.7000	0.9000	0.6000	0.8000	0.3000	0.2000	**0.5700**
P30	0.5000	0.5333	0.5333	0.8000	0.5667	0.8667	0.7000	0.8000	0.1333	0.1000	**0.5533**

retrieval algorithms. However, this implies a significant increase in the workload of the clinicians when handling these datasets.

Although this method was developed for the VISCERAL Retrieval Benchmark tasks and dataset, both the clinical correlations and the general approach for obtaining relevant visual features can be implemented for similar clinical tasks. Nevertheless, the results obtained during the VISCERAL Retrieval Benchmark showed the advantage of combining multimodal information in the search for differential diagnosis medical cases. The semi-automatic method obtained the highest scores for the majority of topics when compared to the other runs submitted in the Benchmark. It includes both textual and visual information in the queries and managed to index a dataset of >2000 medical cases with radiology reports and 3D patient scans.

13.4 Conclusions

A semi-automatic multimodal (using text and visual information) medical case-based retrieval approach is presented. A rule-based weighting of the anatomical and clinical RadLex term correlations from radiology reports is used as a baseline to find useful clinical features from the cases. The results of the processing only text data (RadLex IDs) are further improved with state-of-the-art techniques (Riesz wavelets, image registration and covariance descriptors) to compute a visual similarity score between the medical images in the cases. The method was implemented and tested in the VISCERAL Retrieval Benchmark 2015, with overall promising results for the retrieval of relevant cases for differential medical diagnosis. More work is needed to address the scalability of this approach and the inclusion of new clinical cases.

Acknowledgements This work was supported by the EU in FP7 through VISCERAL (318068), Khresmoi (257528) and the Swiss National National Foundation (SNF grant 205320–141300/1).

References

1. Arsigny V, Fillard P, Pennec X, Ayache N (2006) Log-Euclidean metrics for fast and simple calculus on diffusion tensors. Magn Reson Med 56(2):411–421
2. Cirujeda P, Mateo X, Dicente Y, Binefa X (2014) MCOV: a covariance descriptor for fusion of texture and shape features in 3D point clouds. In: International conference on 3D vision (3DV)
3. Depeursinge A, Foncubierta-Rodriguez A, Ville D, Müller H (2011) Lung texture classification using locally-oriented riesz components. In: Fichtinger G, Martel A, Peters T (eds) MICCAI 2011. LNCS, vol 6893. Springer, Heidelberg, pp 231–238. doi:10.1007/978-3-642-23626-6_29
4. García Seco de Herrera A, Kalpathy-Cramer J, Demner Fushman D, Antani S, Müller H (2013) Overview of the ImageCLEF 2013 medical tasks. In: Working notes of CLEF 2013 (Cross Language Evaluation Forum)
5. García Seco de Herrera A, Foncubierta-Rodríguez A, Müller H (2015) Medical case-based retrieval: integrating query MeSH terms for query-adaptive multi-modal fusion. In: SPIE medical imaging. International Society for Optics and Photonics

6. García Seco de Herrera A, Müller H, Bromuri S (2015) Overview of the ImageCLEF 2015 medical classification task. In: Working notes of CLEF 2015 (Cross Language Evaluation Forum)
7. Hanbury A, Müller H, Langs G, Weber MA, Menze BH, Fernandez TS (2012) Bringing the algorithms to the data: cloud–based benchmarking for medical image analysis. In: Catarci T, Forner P, Hiemstra D, Peñas A, Santucci G (eds) CLEF 2012. LNCS, vol 7488. Springer, Heidelberg, pp 24–29. doi:10.1007/978-3-642-33247-0_3
8. Jiménez del Toro OA, Foncubierta-Rodríguez A, Vargas Gómez MI, Müller H, Depeursinge A (2013) Epileptogenic lesion quantification in MRI using contralateral 3D texture comparisons. In: Mori K, Sakuma I, Sato Y, Barillot C, Navab N (eds) MICCAI 2013. LNCS, vol 8150. Springer, Heidelberg, pp 353–360. doi:10.1007/978-3-642-40763-5_44
9. Jiménez del Toro OA, Foncubierta-Rodríguez A, Depeursinge A, Müller H (2015) Texture classification of anatomical structures in CT using a context-free machine learning approach. In: SPIE medical imaging 2015
10. Jiménez-del-Toro OA, Cirujeda P, Cid YD, Müller H (2015) RadLex terms and local texture features for multimodal medical case retrieval. In: Müller H, Jimenez del Toro OA, Hanbury A, Langs G, Foncubierta Rodríguez A (eds) Multimodal retrieval in the medical domain. LNCS, vol 9059. Springer, Cham, pp 144–152. doi:10.1007/978-3-319-24471-6_14
11. Jiménez-del-Toro OA, Hanbury A, Langs G, Foncubierta–Rodríguez A, Müller H (2015) Overview of the VISCERAL retrieval benchmark 2015. In: Müller H, Jimenez del Toro OA, Hanbury A, Langs G, Foncubierta Rodríguez A (eds) Multimodal retrieval in the medical domain. LNCS, vol 9059. Springer, Cham, pp 115–123. doi:10.1007/978-3-319-24471-6_10
12. Klein S, Pluim JP, Staring M, Viergever MA (2009) Adaptive stochastic gradient descent optimisation for image registration. Int J Comput Vis 81(3):227–239
13. Klein S, Staring M, Murphy K, Viergever MA, Pluim JP (2010) Elastix: a toolbox for intensity-based medical image registration. IEEE Trans Med Imaging 29(1):196–205
14. Kurtz C, Depeursinge A, Napel S, Beaulieu CF, Rubin DL (2014) On combining visual and ontological similarities for medical image retrieval applications. Med Image Anal 18(7):1082–1100
15. Langlotz CP (2006) RadLex: a new method for indexing online educational materials. Radiographics 26(6):1595–1597
16. Langs G, Hanbury A, Menze B, Müller H (2013) VISCERAL: towards large data in medical imaging — challenges and directions. In: Greenspan H, Müller H, Syeda-Mahmood T (eds) MCBR-CDS 2012. LNCS, vol 7723. Springer, Heidelberg, pp 92–98. doi:10.1007/978-3-642-36678-9_9
17. Müller H, Michoux N, Bandon D, Geissbuhler A (2004) A review of content-based image retrieval systems in medicine-clinical benefits and future directions. Int J Med Inform 73(1):1–23
18. Rubin GD (2000) Data explosion: the challenge of multidetector-row CT. Eur J Radiol 36(2):74–80
19. Rubin D, Napel S (2010) Imaging informatics: toward capturing and processing semantic information in radiology images. Yearb Med Inform 2010:34–42
20. Spanier AB, Joskowicz L (2015) Medical case-based retrieval of patient records using the RadLex hierarchical lexicon. In: Müller H, Jimenez del Toro OA, Hanbury A, Langs G, Foncubierta Rodríguez A (eds) Multimodal retrieval in the medical domain. LNCS, vol 9059. Springer, Cham, pp 129–138. doi:10.1007/978-3-319-24471-6_12
21. Unser M, Van De Ville D (2010) Wavelet steerability and the higher-order Riesz transform. IEEE Trans Image Process 19(3):636–652

Chapter 14
Text- and Content-Based Medical Image Retrieval in the VISCERAL Retrieval Benchmark

Fan Zhang, Yang Song, Weidong Cai, Adrien Depeursinge
and Henning Müller

Abstract Text- and content-based retrieval are the most widely used approaches for medical image retrieval. They capture the similarity between the images from different perspectives: text-based methods rely on manual textual annotations or captions associated with images; content-based approaches are based on the visual content of the images themselves such as colours and textures. Text-based retrieval can better meet the high-level expectations of humans but is limited by the time-consuming annotations. Content-based retrieval can automatically extract the visual features for high-throughput processing; however, its performance is less favourable than the text-based approaches due to the gap between low-level visual features and high-level human expectations. In this chapter, we present the participation from our joint research team of USYD/HES-SO in the VISCERAL retrieval task. Five different methods are introduced, of which two are based on the anatomy–pathology terms, two are based on the visual image content and the last one is based on the fusion of the aforementioned methods. The comparison results, given the different methods indicated that the text-based methods outperformed the content-based retrieval and the fusion of text and visual contents, generated the best performance overall.

F. Zhang (✉) · Y. Song · W. Cai
Biomedical and Multimedia Information Technology (BMIT) Research Group,
School of Information Technologies, University of Sydney, Sydney, NSW, Australia
e-mail: fzha8048@uni.sydney.edu.au

W. Cai
e-mail: tom.cai@sydney.edu.au

A. Depeursinge · H. Müller
University of Applied Sciences Western Switzerland (HES-SO), Sierre, Switzerland
e-mail: adrien.depeursinge@hevs.ch

H. Müller
e-mail: henning.mueller@hevs.ch

© The Author(s) 2017
A. Hanbury et al. (eds.), *Cloud-Based Benchmarking
of Medical Image Analysis*, DOI 10.1007/978-3-319-49644-3_14

237

14.1 Introduction

Medical image data produced has been growing rapidly in quantity, content and dimension, due to an enormous increase in the number of diverse clinical examinations performed in digital form and to the large range of image modalities and protocols available [1–5]. Retrieving a set of images that are clinically relevant to the query from a large image database has been the focus of medical research and clinical practice [6–9]. The relevance between the images is normally computed in two manners, i.e. text and content based. The text-based approach is performed given the manual clinical / pathological descriptions, which require that the experts manually index the images with alphanumerical keywords if no text is already available with the images. The content-based retrieval is based on the image visual content information, which automatically extracts the rich visual properties / features to characterize the images [10–12]. While the text-based retrieval is the more common method, the content-based approach is attracting more interest due to the fact that medical image data have expanded rapidly in the past two decades [13, 15–17]. The combination of the two approaches suggests a potential direction of medical image retrieval for performance improvement [18].

In the VISCERAL Retrieval Benchmark, [1]we conducted medical image retrieval based on multimodal and multidimensional data [20]. The similarities between medical cases are computed based on the extracts of the medical records, radiology images and radiology reports. The VISCERAL Retrieval dataset consists of 2311 volumes originated from three different modalities of CT, MRT1 and MRT2. The volumes are from different human body regions such as the abdomen, thorax and the whole body. Within the whole dataset, 1815 volumes are provided with anatomy–pathology terms extracted from the radiology reports. A total of 10 topics with diagnosis and case description were used as queries (see [20] for details). Each of them was annotated with the 3D bounding box of the region of interest (ROI), binary mask of the main organ affected and the corresponding anatomy–pathology terms. A brief introduction of our participation has been reported in [19] and more on the VISCERAL data in general, and the evaluation approach can be found in [20]. Our experimental results are reported with text-based retrieval that utilized the anatomy–pathology terms, with visual content-based retrieval that made use of the visual content features, and with information fusion that combined the above results.

The structure is as follows: in Sect. 14.2, we introduce the text, visual content and fusion retrieval methods that were used in our participation; in Sect. 14.3, we present the experimental results and discussion; and we provide the conclusion in Sect. 14.4.

---

[1]http://www.visceral.eu/benchmarks/retrieval2-benchmark/.

14.2   Methods

A general framework of image retrieval consists of the following steps [13, 14]: feature extraction, similarity calculation and relevance feedback, as illustrated in Fig. 14.1. For our methods, the feature extraction is conducted by analysing the anatomy–pathology term (Sects. 14.2.1 and 14.2.2) and the image content information (Sect. 14.2.3). The similarity is computed by measuring the Euclidean distance between the feature vectors. The relevance feedback is extracted based on the neighbourhood information among the cases for retrieval result refinement (Sect. 14.2.4).

14.2.1   Term Weighting Retrieval

Medical image retrieval is conventionally performed with text-based approaches, which rely on manual annotation with alphanumerical keywords. The anatomy–pathology term files provided in the VISCERAL Retrieval Benchmark list the pathology terms and affected anatomies that were extracted from the German radiology reports and mapped to RadLex. The co-occurence of different anatomy–pathology terms on the same cases can be used to evaluate the terms' effectiveness of finding the similarity between subjects, for example, of some "stop words" that occur widely but have little influence on describing the similarities. Our text-based methods are based on the co-occurrence matrix between the terms and cases.

For our first text-based method, we used term frequency inverse document (case) frequency (TF-IDF) [21] to weight the terms for each case. TF-IDF can find the rare terms that carry more information than the frequent ones and is thus widely applied in term weighting problems. Formally, a case-term co-occurrence matrix $OCC_{NT \times NC}$ is constructed according to the anatomy–pathology terms on different cases, where the element $occ(t, c)$ refers to the number of occurrences of term T_t on case C_c,

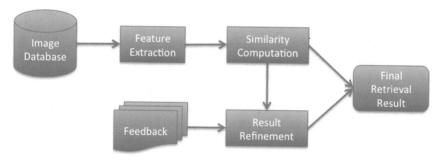

Fig. 14.1 Image retrieval pipeline in this study: (1) feature extraction from the anatomy–pathology terms and image content information; (2) similarity computation to measure the similarity between the cases in terms of feature vectors; (3) result refinement to rerank the candidate cases according to the feedbacks extracted from the neighbourhood information among the cases

NC is the number of cases and NT is the number of terms. Term frequency $TF(t, c)$ evaluates the frequency of the term T_t occurred on the case C_c, which is

$$TF(t, c) = \frac{occ(t, c)}{\sum_{t \in [1, NT]} occ(t, c)}. \tag{14.1}$$

Inverse document (case) frequency $IDF(t)$ indicates whether the term T_t is common or rare across all cases, which is

$$IDF(t) = \log(\frac{\sum_{c \in [1, NC]} occ(t, c)}{1 + occ(t, c)}). \tag{14.2}$$

TF-IDF measure of T_t for C_c is then computed as

$$TF\text{-}IDF(t, c) = TF(t, c) \times IDF(t). \tag{14.3}$$

Case C_c is finally formulated as a vector of TF-IDF measures of all terms as

$$V_{TF\text{-}IDF}(c) = (TF\text{-}IDF(1, c), ..., TF\text{-}IDF(NT, c)). \tag{14.4}$$

The Euclidean distance between the vectors is then computed. We conducted a k-NN method for retrieval, which means selecting the cases that have the closest feature vectors to the one of the queries $V_{TF\text{-}IDF}(q)$ in terms of Euclidean distance.

14.2.2 Semantics Retrieval

While the TF-IDF method merely utilizes the direct co-occurrence relationship between the terms and cases, this relationship can be further used to infer the semantic information and can provide a more discriminative description of these terms for similarity computation. The latent semantic topic model is one of the most representative methods that can automatically extract the semantic information based on the co-occurrence relationship. It assumes that each image can be considered as a mixture of latent topics, and the latent topic is a probability distribution of terms. In this study, we applied probabilistic latent semantic analysis (pLSA) [22], which is a widely used latent topic extraction technique, for learning the latent semantics.

The schema of pLSA is shown in Fig. 14.2. pLSA considers that the observed probability of a term T_t occurring on a case C_c can be expressed with a latent or unobserved set of latent topics $Z = \{z_h | h \in [1, H]\}$, where H is the number of latent topics, as:

$$P(t|c) = \sum_h P(t|z_h) \cdot P(z_h|c). \tag{14.5}$$

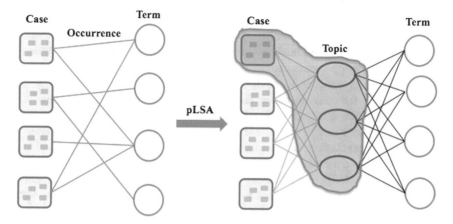

Fig. 14.2 Latent topic generation with pLSA

The probability $P(z_h|c)$ describes the distribution of latent topics given a certain case. The latent topics Z can be learnt by fitting the model with the expectation–maximization (EM) [25] algorithm that maximizes the likelihood function L:

$$L = \prod_t \prod_c P(t|c)^{occ(t,c)}. \tag{14.6}$$

After the latent topic extraction, each case is represented as the probability vector of the extracted latent topics,

$$V_{pLSA}(c) = (P(z_1|c), ..., P(z_H|c)), \tag{14.7}$$

where each element is the probability of the latent topic given this case. The similarity between different cases is then measured by the Euclidean distance between the probability vectors, followed by the k-NN method for retrieval as introduced in Sect. 14.2.1. During the experiments, we empirically fixed the number of latent topics to 20, i.e. $H = 20$.

14.2.3   BoVW Retrieval

Unlike the aforementioned text-based methods, the visual content-based retrieval computes the similarity between the images based on their visual characteristics, such as the texture and colour. In the literature, there are many methods that can automatically extract the visual features to characterize the medical images [2, 26–28]. The Bag of Visual Words (BoVW) [29, 30] method, which is one of the popular methods for visual content-based image retrieval, is applied as our first content-based retrieval method. The BoVW model represents an image with a visual word frequency histogram that is obtained by assigning the local visual features to the closest visual words in the dictionary. Rather than matching the visual feature descriptors directly, the BoVW-based approaches compare the images according to the visual words that are assumed to have higher discriminative power [29].

Specifically, the scale invariant feature transform (SIFT) [31] descriptors are extracted from the image to obtain a collection of local patch features for each image/case. The entire patch feature set computed from all images in the database is then grouped into clusters, e.g. with k-means method. Each cluster is regarded as a visual word W, and the whole cluster collection is considered as the visual dictionary $D = \{W_d | d \in [1, ND]\}$, where ND is the size of dictionary. Following that, all patch features in one image are assigned to the visual words, generating a visual word frequency histogram to represent this image (case) as,

$$V_{BoVW}(c) = (fre(1, c), ..., fre(ND, c)),\qquad(14.8)$$

where $fre(d, c)$ is the frequency of visual word W_d on case C_c. Finally, the similarity between images is computed based on these frequency histograms for retrieval.

In our experiments, the SIFT [31] descriptors were extracted from each scan of the 3D volume from the axial view. A visual dictionary of size 100, i.e. $ND = 100$ that could be sufficient for capturing local visual details and does not introduce too much noise based on our previous study in medical image analysis [23, 24], was computed with k-means. During the retrieval, given the ROI of a query case, we traversed all possible subregions (of the same size as the ROI in terms of the pixels) in a candidate volume in sliding window manner. Two subregions can be overlapped with an interval of 10 pixels at X/Y/Z directions. The subregion that has the smallest Euclidean distance from the query ROI in terms of visual word frequency histograms was regarded as the most similar area of the candidate to the query ROI, while the other subregions were not used. The distance between the two regions represented the similarity between the query and candidate images in our study. The k-NN method was applied for retrieval considering the obtained similarities.

14.2.4   Retrieval Result Refinement

While the first two steps form a basic retrieval process, relevance feedback refines the retrieval results if the top-ranked items are not fully satisfactory. Relevance feedback is based on the preferences upon the initial retrieval results, which can be provided by the users. However, providing manual feedback can be quite challenging due to the huge amount of image data. The relevance can also be affected since manual interpretation sometimes could be error-prone. The neighbourhood among images on the other hand can be used as a form of relevance feedback and is expected to be beneficial for image retrieval.

Algorithm 1 Pseudo code for preference and relativity computation

---

Input: Number of iterations T, neighborhood matrix A.
Output: Preference and relativity values.
1: **initialize** $rel_0 = 1$ and $pref_0 = 1$.
2: **for** each it in $[1, IT]$ **do**
3:   **for** each C_{cr} **do**
4:     Compute $pref_{it}(C_{cr})$ based on $rel_{it-1}(C_{cc})$ using Eq.(14.9);
5:   **end for**;
6:   **for** each C_{cc} **do**
7:     Compute $rel_{it}(C_{cc})$ based on $pref_{it}(C_{cr})$ using Eq.(14.10);
8:   **end for**;
9:   $L2$-normalize $pref_{it}$ of all retrieved items.
10:   $L2$-normalize rel_{it} of all candidates.
11: **end for**;
12: **return** $pref_{it}$ and rel_{it}.

Based on the results of the BoVW method, we further conducted a retrieval result refinement process based on our recent work [32]. In our method, we assume that the similarity relationship between the initial retrieved results and the remaining candidates can be used as a relevance feedback for result refinement. For a given query image, we first get a ranked list of initial retrieval results based on the BoVW model. Then, the similarities between the retrieved items and all candidates are used to evaluate their *preference* and *relativity*.

Formally, a preference score $pref(C_{cr})$ for the retrieved item C_{cr} is defined to evaluate the preference upon C_{cr} with regard to the query, i.e. relevance and irrelevance. A relativity score $rel(C_{cc})$ is appointed to the candidate image C_{cc}, indicating the similarity of C_{cc} to the query. The two values are computed conditioned on each other regarding the query case C_{cq}: the relativity score $rel(C_{cc})$ of C_{cc} would be high if it is similar to the highly preferred retrieved item C_{cr}, and the preference score $pref(C_{cr})$ of C_{cr} would be high if it is close to the more relevant candidate C_{cc}. The relativity score of C_{cc} is formulated as the sum of preference scores of its neighbouring retrieved items, similar to the preference score of C_{cr}. Denoting rel and $pref$ as the vectors of relativity and preference scores, we have the following formulations:

$$pref(C_{cr}) = \sum_{C_{cc}:A(C_{cc},C_{cr})=1} rel(C_{cc}), \tag{14.9}$$

$$rel(C_{cc}) = \sum_{C_{cr}:A(C_{cc},C_{cr})=1} pref(C_{cr}), \tag{14.10}$$

where A is a matrix indicating the bipartite neighbourhood relationship between the retrieved items and the candidates, i.e. $A(C_{cc}, C_{cr}) = 1$ if C_{cc} is the neighbour of C_{cr}; otherwise, $A(C_{cc}, C_{cr}) = 0$. Equation (14.9) and (14.10) can be alternatively solved iteratively to obtain the relativity and preference scores as shown in Algorithm 1.

We then ranked all candidate images based on their relativity scores, in which the top-ranked ones were regarded as the most similar cases to the query. For our experiments, we selected the top 30 volumes based on the BoVW outputs as the initial results C_{cr}. Then, a bipartite relationship between the initial results C_{cr} and the remaining candidates C_{cc}, which represented the neighbourhood, was constructed by keeping the top 30 candidates for each initial result. The iterative ranking method [32] was applied to recompute the similarity score of each candidate with an iteration number IT of 20, after which the relativity and preference scores tended to be stable and have insignificant influence on the ranking orders of the candidates.

14.2.5 Fusion Retrieval

It is often suggested that the combination of textual and visual features can improve the retrieval performance [18]. Many fusion strategies have been proposed in the past such as maximum combination [34], sum combination [34] and Condorcet fusion [35].

Given the results from the text- and content-based retrievals, we conducted the fusion retrieval by using the sum combination method, which has been effective for textual and visual feature fusion [33]. To do this, a normalization step was firstly incorporated to normalize the similarity scores obtained from the aforementioned results, as:

$$S' = \frac{S - S_{min}}{S_{max} - S_{min}}, \tag{14.11}$$

where S_{min} and S_{max} are the lowest and highest similarity scores obtained within a certain method. The sum combination was then adopted to compute a fusion score for each candidate, as:

$$S_F = \sum_{r \in [1,4]} S'_r, \tag{14.12}$$

where $r \in [1, 4]$ represents the first four methods. The ones with the higher scores were for the results of fusion retrieval.

14.3 Results and Discussion

To evaluate the performance of retrieval results, medical experts were invited to perform relevance assessment of the top-ranked cases for each run. Various evaluation measures were used considering the top-ranked X cases, including the precision for top-ranked 10 and 30 cases (P@10, P@30), mean uninterpolated average precision (MAP), bpref measure and the R-precision.

Figure 14.3 displays the retrieval result for each of the topics given the aforementioned measures. The performances were diverse across the cases. It can be generally observed that better results were obtained for topics 1 and 7 when compared to the

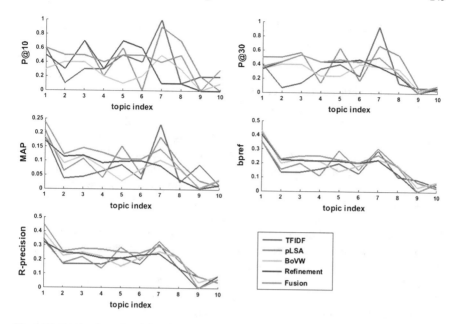

Fig. 14.3 Retrieval results of the 10 topics given different evaluation measures

Table 14.1 Average results of the different measures across the 10 queries

	P@10	P@30	MAP	bpref
TFIDF	0.370	0.277	0.081	0.162
pLSA	0.410	**0.380**	0.094	0.183
BoVW	0.250	0.283	0.078	0.190
Refinement	0.330	0.330	0.083	0.188
Fusion	**0.420**	0.353	**0.110**	**0.207**
Text	0.570	0.497	0.194	0.322
Image	0.330	0.330	0.083	0.188
Mixed	0.688	0.638	0.283	0.340

other topics, but the results for topics 9 and 10 were unfavourable. The differences were due to the different affected regions. Our methods computed the similarity between cases using the entire volumes, instead of focusing on the local details. Therefore, for cases that have relatively smaller annotated regions (the 3D bounding box of the ROI) compared to the others, e.g. case 10, the retrieval performance tended to be less favourable.

Table 14.1 shows the average results of the measures across the 10 queries, with the first five rows from our results and the last three rows showing the best results from all participants of the VISCERAL retrieval benchmark. Within our text-based approaches, pLSA generated better performance when compared to the

TF-IDF method, by further using the latent semantic information inferred from the co-occurrence relationship between cases and terms. Regarding the content-based retrieval, we obtained better results when applying the result refinement. Across the four methods, better performance was obtained from the text-based retrieval when compared to the content-based retrieval. The content-based methods use the visual content characteristics that may have large variation between the relevant cases but small difference between the irrelevant ones. The SIFT feature used in our experiments is widely known for capturing the local image content information, but it sometimes can be hard for SIFT to recognize the subtle visual difference between different images. In addition, while the size of the dictionary was set to 100 in our experiments, it can be varied for different datasets and potentially affect the retrieval performance. The text-based approaches on the other hand compare the different cases directly based on the pathology terms and affected anatomies. Thus, the text-based retrieval obtained the more favourable retrieval results. While the anatomy–pathology terms provide an overall description for the similarity computation, the visual content feature can better capture the local anatomical differences between cases. Therefore, the fusion approach achieved the overall best result, which is in accordance with the findings in the literature. Regarding the comparisons across all VISCERAL Retrieval Benchmark participations, we had the best performance with the result refinement among all image-based methods. The results from the text and fusion methods were less favourable since only co-occurrence information between the terms were used. Further analysis of the terms in the benchmark relating to the entire anatomy–pathology RadLex term collection would be helpful for retrieval improvements.

14.4   Conclusion

In this chapter, we introduced the approaches from our joint research team of USYD/HES-SO to address the VISCERAL Retrieval Benchmark, including the TF-IDF and pLSA methods for text-based retrieval, the BoVW and its result refinement for content-based retrieval, and the fusion retrieval of the above methods. The experimental results are in accordance with the findings in the literature, i.e. the text-based approaches typically perform better than purely visual content-based methods, and the combination of text- and content-based retrieval can achieve improved retrieval performance.

A further potential exploration could be the parameter selection. In this study, we empirically selected the settings of the parameters based on our previous work on other medical image retrieval tasks, such as the number of topics in the semantic retrieval, the size of dictionary in the BoVW retrieval and the number of initial retrieved items in the retrieval result refinement. It would be interesting to learn the parameters within the VISCERAL Retrieval Benchmark dataset but can be difficult due to the large amount of image data and the current lack of ground truth annotations. Another direction can be investigating a better way to combine the textual and image content information. While the fusion retrieval tended to generate better performance in our study in general, we can also observe that the semantic retrieval overperformed the fusion method, e.g. the precision for top-ranked 30 cases (P@30). We expected a better performance if the feature extraction could utilize both textual- and image-content information rather than analysing them individually.

References

1. Doi K (2006) Diagnostic imaging over the last 50 years: research and development in medical imaging science and technology. Phys Med Biol 51:R5–R27
2. Müller H, Michoux N, Bandon D, Geissbuhler A (2004) A review of content-based image retrieval systems in medicine—clinical benefits and future directions. Int J Med Inf 73:1–23
3. Cai W, Feng D, Fulton R (2000) Content-based retrieval of dynamic PET functional images. IEEE Trans Inf Technol Biomed 4(2):152–158
4. Song Y, Cai W, Eberl S, Fulham MJ, Feng D (2011) Thoracic image case retrieval with spatial and contextual information. In: IEEE international symposium biomedical imaging (ISBI), pp 1885–1888
5. Kumar A, Kim J, Cai W, Fulham M, Feng D (2013) Content-based medical image retrieval: a survey of applications to multidimensional and multimodality data. J Digit Imaging 26(6):1025–1039
6. Zhang S, Yang M, Cour T, Yu K, Metaxas D (2014) Query specific rank fusion for image retrieval. IEEE Trans Pattern Anal Mach Intell 47(4):803–815
7. Müller H, Antoine R, Arnaud G, Jean-Paul V, Antoine G (2005) Benefits of content-based visual data access in radiology 1. Radiographics 25(3):849–858
8. Song Y, Cai W, Zhou Y, Wen L, Feng D (2013) Pathology-centric medical image retrieval with hierarchical contextual spatial descriptor. In: IEEE international symposium on biomedical imaging (ISBI), pp 202–205
9. Song Y, Cai W, Eberl S, Fulham MJ, Feng D (2010) A content-based image retrieval framework for multi-modality lung images. In: IEEE international symposium on computer-based medical systems (CBMS), pp 285–290
10. El-Naqa I, Yang Y, Galatsanos NP, Nishikawa RM, Wernick MN (2004) A similarity learning approach to content-based image retrieval: application to digital mammography. IEEE Trans Med Imaging 23:1233–1244
11. Zhang F, Song Y, Cai W, Lee M-Z, Zhou Y, Huang H, Shan S, Fulham MJ, Feng D (2014) Lung nodule classification with multi-level patch-based context analysis. IEEE Trans Biomed Eng 61(4):1155–1166
12. Foncubierta-Rodríguez A, Depeursinge A, Müller H (2012) Using multiscale visual words for lung texture classification and retrieval. In: Müller H, Greenspan H, Syeda-Mahmood T (eds) MCBR-CDS 2011. LNCS, vol 7075. Springer, Heidelberg, pp 69–79. doi:10.1007/978-3-642-28460-1_7
13. Cai W, Kim J, Feng D (2008) Content-based medical image retrieval. Elsevier book section 4:83–113
14. Squire D, Müller W, Müller H, Raki J (1999) Content-based query of image databases, inspirations from text retrieval: inverted files, frequency-based weights and relevance feedback. In: The 11th scandinavian conference on image analysis, pp 143–149
15. Müller H, Deserno TM (2011) Content-based medical image retrieval. In: Deserno TM (ed) Biomedical image processing. Springer, Berlin, pp 471–494
16. Haas S, Donner R, Burner A, Holzer M, Langs G (2012) Superpixel-based interest points for effective bags of visual words medical image retrieval. In: Müller H, Greenspan H, Syeda-Mahmood T (eds) MCBR-CDS 2011. LNCS, vol 7075. Springer, Heidelberg, pp 58–68. doi:10.1007/978-3-642-28460-1_6

17. Zhang F, Song Y, Cai W, Hauptmann AG, Liu S, Liu SQ, Feng DD, Chen M (2015) Ranking-based vocabulary pruning in bag-of-features for image retrieval. In: Chalup SK, Blair AD, Randall M (eds) ACALCI 2015. LNCS (LNAI), vol 8955. Springer, Cham, pp 436–445. doi:10. 1007/978-3-319-14803-8_34

18. Müller H, Kalpathy-Cramer J (2010) The ImageCLEF medical retrieval task at ICPR 2010 — information fusion to combine visual and textual information. In: Ünay D, Çataltepe Z, Aksoy S (eds) ICPR 2010. LNCS, vol 6388. Springer, Heidelberg, pp 99–108. doi:10.1007/978-3-642-17711-8_11

19. Zhang F, Song Y, Cai W, Depeursinge A, Müller H (2015) USYD/HES-SO in the VISCERAL retrieval benchmark. In: Müller H, Jimenez del Toro OA, Hanbury A, Langs G, Foncubierta Rodríguez A (eds) Multimodal retrieval in the medical domain. LNCS, vol 9059. Springer, Cham, pp 139–143. doi:10.1007/978-3-319-24471-6_13

20. Hanbury A, Müller H, Langs G, Weber MA, Menze BH, Fernandez TS (2012) Bringing the algorithms to the data: cloud–based benchmarking for medical image analysis. In: Catarci T, Forner P, Hiemstra D, Peñas A, Santucci G (eds) CLEF 2012. LNCS, vol 7488. Springer, Heidelberg, pp 24–29. doi:10.1007/978-3-642-33247-0_3

21. Jones KS (1972) A statistical interpretation of term specificity and its application in retrieval. J Doc 28:11–21

22. Hofmann T (2001) Unsupervised learning by probabilistic latent semantic analysis. Mach Learn 42:177–196

23. Zhang F, Song Y, Cai W, Liu S, Liu S, Pujol S, Kikinis R (2016) ADNI: pairwise latent semantic association for similarity computation in medical imaging. IEEE Trans Biomed Eng 63(5):1058–1069

24. Zhang F, Song Y, Cai W, Hauptmann AG, Liu S, Pujol S, Kikinis R, Chen M (2016) Dictionary pruning with visual word significance for medical image retrieval. Neurocomputing 177:75–88

25. Heinrich G (2005) Parameter estimation for text analysis. Technical report

26. Zhang X, Liu W, Dundar M, Badve S, Zhang S (2015) Towards large scale histopathological image analysis: hashing-based image retrieval. IEEE Trans Med Imaging 34:496–506

27. Yang W, Lu Z, Yu M, Huang M, Feng Q, Chen W (2012) Content-based retrieval of focal liver lesions using bag-of-visual-words representations of single- and multiphase contrast-enhanced CT images. J Digit Imaging 25:708–719

28. Song Y, Cai W, Eberl S, Fulham MJ, Feng D (2011) Thoracic image matching with appearance and spatial distribution. In: The 33rd annual international conference of the IEEE engineering in medicine and biology society (EMBC), pp 4469–4472

29. Sivic J, Zisserman A (2003) Video Google: a text retrieval approach to object matching in videos. In: IEEE international conference on computer vision (ICCV), pp 1470–1477

30. Liu S, Cai W, Song Y, Pujol S, Kikinis R, Feng D (2013) A bag of semantic words model for medical content-based retrieval. In: The 16th international conference on MICCAI workshop on medical content-based retrieval for clinical decision support

31. Lowe DG (1999) Object recognition from local scale-invariant features. In: IEEE international conference on computer vision (ICCV), pp 1150–1157

32. Cai W, Zhang F, Song Y, Liu S, Wen L, Eberl S, Fulham M, Feng D (2014) Automated feedback extraction for medical imaging retrieval. In: IEEE international symposium on biomedical imaging (ISBI), pp 907–910

33. Zhou X, Depeursinge A, Müller H (2010) Information fusion for combining visual and textual image retrieval. In: International conference on pattern recognition (ICPR), pp 1590–1593

34. Fox EA, Shaw JA (1993) Combination of multiple searches. Text retrieval conference, pp 243–252

35. Montague M, Aslam JA (2002) Condorcet fusion for improved retrieval. In: Proceedings of the eleventh international conference on information and knowledge management (CIKM), pp 538–548

Index

Printed in the United States
By Bookmasters